AF506181

THE MONITORING SOURCEBOOK

VOLUME 2

NURSING PRACTICE

CATHERINE DEVET, RN, MSN, EdD

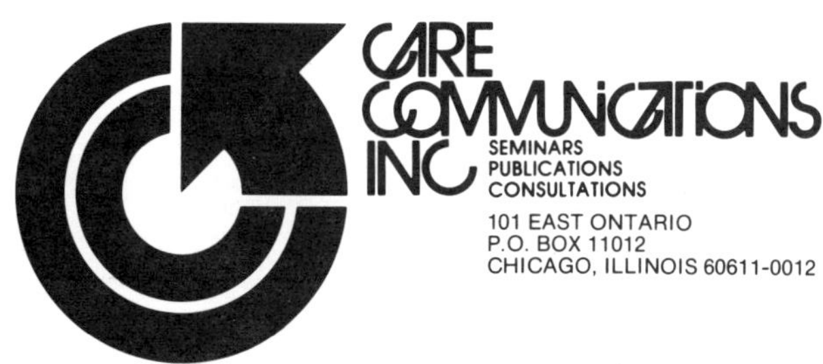

101 EAST ONTARIO
P.O. BOX 11012
CHICAGO, ILLINOIS 60611-0012

ACKNOWLEDGEMENTS

The author gratefully acknowledges the extensive contributions, encouragement and support given by:

- **Eric D. Joseph, MPH,** Director of Research and Development, Care Communications, Inc.

- **Gerry Stearns, MSPH,** President, Care Communications, Inc.

In addition, the following registered nurses provided valuable information and assistance:

- **Betty Lou Miccio, BS,** Vice President and Director, Professional Practice and Quality Assurance, New Jersey Hospital Association

- **Gerry Svendson, MS,** Associate Hospital Director of Patient Care, R.E. Thomason General Hospital, El Paso, TX

- **Andrea Edge, MBA,** Director of Nursing, Peralta Hospital, Oakland, CA

- **Mary Ann Zettelmaier, MSN,** Nurse Consultant, Maternal-Infant Health, Chesterton, IN

- **Mary Beth Nienstedt, MN,** Clinical Nurse Specialist and **Deborah S. Briggs,** Administrative Director, Emergency and Trauma Center, Borgess Medical Center, Kalamazoo, MI

- **Mary Ratliff, MSN,** Director, Critical Care Nursing Department; **Joyce French, MSN,** Director, Maternal-Child Health Department; **Patricia A. Cornell, MN,** Head Nurse, Young Adults and Pediatric Critical Care; and **Sue Drenth, BSN,** Head Nurse, Pediatrics, Blodgett Memorial Medical Center, Grand Rapids, MI

- **Janice Kinsey, BSN,** Quality Assurance Coordinator - Nursing, Edward W. Sparrow Hospital, Lansing, MI

EDITOR: Karen Sandrick

COVER DESIGN: Julie Koenig

PRODUCTION AND LAYOUT: Kathleen Gletis
Karl Weller
Cathy Kodelsky
Lauretta Romanoski

Second Edition Copyright © 1987
First Edition Copyright © 1984

Care Communications, Inc.
101 East Ontario
Chicago, IL 60611

International Standard Book Number: 0-916499-32-4

THE MONITORING SOURCEBOOK
VOLUME 2
NURSING PRACTICE

Chapter	Title	Page
1	Creating a Nursing Data Base Through Monitoring	1
2	Perspectives on Monitoring	11
3	The Structure of a Monitor	17
4	Types and Categories of Monitors	29
5	Integrating the Monitoring Activity into the "80-Hour Week"	63
6	Choosing Topics for Monitors	71
7	Choosing High-Priority Topics	99
8	Completing the Specifications for Monitors	107
9	Completing an Agenda of Department Monitors	125
10	Topics for Monitors for Specific Clinical Areas	163
	Bibliography	207
	Worksheets	211

1: Creating a Nursing Data Base Through Monitoring

Once considered only an adjunct to medicine, nursing has emerged as a profession firmly grounded in its own scientific theory and accountable to society for the independent judgments and therapeutic interventions of its practitioners. As nursing practice has grown more complicated and sophisticated, so have the demands on nurse managers and their staff. These demands arise from the nursing profession itself, regulatory and accrediting agencies, such as the Joint Commission on Accreditation of Hospitals (JCAH), American Osteopathic Association (AOA) and hospitals, which are facing not only an economic crisis but an increasingly unfavorable malpractice climate.

Because the nursing department serves as the fulcrum for all patient care activities within a hospital, the extent to which it can meet the challenges posed by these various entities significantly influences the contribution that nursing makes to the hospital in its struggle to survive the turbulent changes in the health care market place.

In their attempts to adapt to the internal and external demands that are being placed on nursing practice, nurse managers have initiated numerous efforts to gather pertinent data on the effects that nursing services have on the utilization and quality of patient care services. Unfortunately, these efforts have often produced a fragmented, incomplete or erroneous picture of the services provided by the nursing department. Today's nurse managers realize that they can no longer afford to maintain divisive and competing evaluation activities. They recognize the need for a coherent, integrated and complete Nursing Data Base on the many critical issues that they must address each day, including:

- Utilization of nursing services

- Staff performance of patient care functions

- Provision of a safe environment for patients, visitors and staff

- Thorough documentation of nursing practice

- Quality assurance in an environment of scarce resources

- Risk management

The integrity of the nursing department and the survival of the hospital hinge on nurse managers' and their staff's ability to work cooperatively to engineer a common and complete data base that effectively meets a variety of crucial needs. This formal data base can be created through a *comprehensive* and *systematic monitoring system* that generates the data needed by nurse managers and guides them in their use of data to make sound decisions regarding the present operation and future direction of the department and the hospital. The purpose of this book is to present nurse managers with a system they can use to move confidently toward meeting the many responsibilities that are being pressed upon them.

Professional Responsibilities of Nurse Managers

Nursing is the only health care profession that is universally expected to complete a complex process for every patient for whom it is responsible. Nurses must:

- Assess patients

- Make timely nursing diagnoses

- Establish appropriate goals and a plan of care

- Implement pertinent interventions

- Evaluate the success of the nursing process and revise the process when necessary

The nursing process has been recognized as the basis for nursing practice by regulatory and accrediting agencies, legislatures and the courts. Nurses are mandated to effectively use the nursing process in the care of their patients by JCAH, AOA, American Nurses' Association (ANA), state nurse practice acts and judicial decisions. Nurse managers consequently must assure that nurses are correctly performing each step in the process and thoroughly documenting the effects of nursing care on patient outcomes. Through monitoring, nurse managers can obtain a permanent record of the professional activities that were performed and patients' responses to them.

In addition to confirming the appropriate use of the nursing process, the profession is expected to assure that its practitioners have achieved and continue to maintain recognized levels of expertise. This expertise includes skill in performing standard protocols and procedures, the proper use and care of equipment and supplies and the maintenance of a safe environment for patients, visitors and colleagues. Nurse managers must assess the extent to which the staff meet these responsibilities to spot and correct in a timely manner substandard performance or wasteful use of resources. Monitors that use a framework of the department's standards of care allow nurse managers to review and document staff performance of all aspects of nursing practice.

Responsibilities of Nurse Managers in a Cost Containment Era

Prospective pricing systems and other efforts to reduce health care expenditures have precipitated an economic crisis in hospitals across the country. Nursing, as the core of the acute care institution, holds the key to the financial viability of the hospital. The nursing department has, after all, the largest number of personnel and a high concentration of professional staff. Its provision of professional services in a cost-effective manner therefore is essential to the fiscal health of the institution.

However, since nurse managers in the past have concentrated on the clinical performance of the department and not the cost of this clinical performance, they have not focused on budgetary matters, productivity of staff, profitability of services or other issues related to the cost-effective delivery of nursing care.

The new reimbursement systems also have centered attention on the costs of nursing services. With the previous cost-based method of paying for hospital care, there was little need to itemize charges for nursing services. Nursing care was simply made part of the "room and board" charges on a patient's bill. Now that payment for hospital care progressively is being based on preestablished flat rates, hospital administrators, chief financial officers and nurse managers are carefully analyzing the cost of performing specific nursing functions. This infusion of economic concerns into the complex world of providing clinical services has placed a number of new pressures on nurse managers.

One such pressure is the increased responsibility of nurse managers to create, implement and manage a budget that conforms to the diminished financial resources available to the hospital. The nursing department must no longer be viewed strictly as a cost center with its budget regulated by non-nursing administrators as it has been in the past. Nurse managers must plan budgets properly using monitors to track the nursing services rendered to patients and determine the actual costs of delivering those services so appropriate charges for the department's services can be made.

Because the reimbursement a hospital receives is currently dependent upon the case-mix of the patient groups it serves, nurse managers are under pressure to become knowledgeable about the case-mix of their institution. In particular, they must learn what costs are incurred by specific groups of patients and how nursing services contribute to these costs. For a high volume or unprofitable case-mix group, nurse managers need to establish monitors that can identify inappropriate or costly nursing services that substantially increase the cost of care but do not significantly affect the quality of care or the patient's outcome.

Since the costs of nursing services are intimately linked to the productivity of nursing personnel, nurse managers cannot adequately address the true costs of nursing services without determining how nurses are utilized and what productivity levels they are achieving. These measures are essential to support the number and mix of personnel nurse managers believe are necessary for delivering quality patient care. These measures also are useful for demonstrating the degree to which nurses perform non-nursing functions when personnel from other departments are unavailable. The data can then be used to negotiate with appropriate departments about who should be responsible for performing these functions or what adjustments should be made in the nursing budget to compensate the department for performing these extra duties.

As hospital administrators feel increasing financial pressure due to declines in patient census, they will search for ways to cut the costs of operation. A traditional method for reducing expenditures is to reduce staff. Although the census and lengths of stay within hospitals have been declining, patients' acuity levels and the intensity of nursing services needed have been increasing. With the aging of the American society, caring for more elderly persons with chronic as well as acute conditions will become more common. Nurse managers must closely monitor changes in the acuity and complexity of patient conditions so they can objectively support staffing levels that cannot be justified by census numbers alone. Nurse managers must justify the allocation of scarce resources to their department based on data that demonstrate patients' need for resources and the impact on the quality of patient care that staff reductions will have.

The profitability of services provided by the hospital is a vital concern as the institution strives to not only "break even" but procure capital to improve services and obtain the technology that is needed for providing high quality patient care. The nursing department is integral to the profitability of hospital services. The quality of patient care delivered by nurses can decrease patients' length of stay and their complication rates and thereby improve the hospital's profit picture. Nursing care also has a great deal to do with the satisfaction of patients, visitors and physicians with hospitalization, which can affect admission rates to the institution. Nurse managers can use data from monitors to illustrate the effect that nursing care has on the hospital's financial performance by documenting the efficiency of performance of the nursing staff, the satisfaction of users of nursing services and the decline of untoward adverse incidents.

The pressure resulting from competition among health care providers may be an uncomfortable reality for nurse managers, but an institution's survival may depend on the innovative and progressive "products" that the nursing department can market successfully. The nursing department, with its diversity of services and concentration of professionals, provides many marketable services. Nurse managers need to institute monitors that can help identify which "products" can be offered by the department and then help evaluate the success of these "products" as they are developed and implemented.

Responsibilities of Nurse Managers in Ethical Issues

Although ethical issues have always been of concern to the nursing profession, nurse managers and their staffs are more likely to face ethical dilemmas in the future because of the rapid advance of expensive technologies in a cost-containment era. In the past, if a piece of equipment or service was believed to be necessary to improve the quality of care, that belief was sufficient to warrant its monetary support. This perspective has been replaced by the beliefs that "more is not necessarily better," that the quality of a person's life as well as its length are important considerations in health care decisions and that the present cost trends in health care will bankrupt some of its major purchasers (ie, Social Security) in the next few years. These changes in attitude have raised, and will continue to raise, serious questions about equal access to patient care, discrimination in the delivery of services to patient populations based on age or payor status and the use of expensive technologies for the benefit of a few patients while inadequate or reduced services are given to many.

Answers to these sensitive ethical issues will be slow, imperfect and painful. To help assess the issues objectively, nurse managers and staff must plan monitors that will provide information on the efficacy of treatment modalities and the effect on patient outcomes when certain treatments are restricted.

Responsibilities of Nurse Managers in Risk Management

Given the tremendous diversity of expectations associated with nurses' provision of quality care in an environment of restricted resources, it is not surprising that nursing has become a vital component of effective risk management efforts in hospitals. Monitoring risk management concerns in the nursing services is becoming critical as hospitals strive to meet the growing number of malpractice claims against them. Although nurses can be held individually accountable for their negligent acts and they are being named as defendants in malpracice cases more frequently, they often are not at financial risk. At the present time, hospitals bear the financial consequences of malpractice and negligence suits involving the quality of nursing care that has been rendered. When financial resources are diverted to litigation and the award of damages, the hospital has fewer resources available to meet operational needs, purchase capital equipment and improve employees' salaries. Identifying and rectifying deficiencies in nursing practice can significantly reduce the potential for harm for patients, visitors or staff and a resultant law suit as well as prevent financial loss.

In summary, modern nurse managers must cope with multiple responsibilites that affect the very survival of their profession and the hospital in which they work. Because they are now accountable for both the quality and the costs of their department's services, nurse managers must not only ensure that the nursing department:

- Maintains the quality of services

- Meets increasingly stringent standards of care set by regulatory bodies, accrediting agencies and professional organizations.

- Identifies and solves problems that may expose the hospital and its staff to liability

They must also ensure that their department:

- Uses resources appropriately

- Operates profitably

- Reduces costs wherever possible

- Develops services that will help the hospital remain competitive

To meet these responsibilities, nurse managers must discard the disjointed systems of data collection and utilization of the past. They must create a data base that demonstrates the importance of nursing services to the hospital's delivery of high quality health care and that serves to protect the hospital against losses—losses of money, technical capability and status within the health care delivery system and the community.

Components of the Nursing Data Base

Because many hospital administrators have been developing data bases that address quality, cost, risk management and productivity for all departments, contemporary nurse managers have many data resources within their department and in other departments as well.

Nurse managers cannot possibly collect, screen or evaluate *all* available data on the performance and utilization of their clinical areas and in the department. Nor can they merely speculate about the kinds of information that can be of value to them, their staff and the hospital administration. Instead, nurse managers must carefully plan the data that will be generated within their department and anticipate the data that must be requested from sources outside the department. They must be extremely selective in the process and try to identify the information that will have the biggest "payoff" for the department and the hospital.

To start planning a realistic as well as a comprehensive nursing data base, nurse managers must first define precisely the purposes for which data are collected and reviewed. Data may be gathered to:

- More accurately estimate the demands for nursing services by physicians, other departments and various patient groups

- Identify or verify problems in the clinical appropriateness and timeliness of demands for service

- Demonstrate the need for changing the nature, timing and frequency of services offered by the department to enhance the quality, efficiency or profitability of departmental services

- Determine whether other clinicians' use the results of tests and recommendations appropriately

- Judge how well staff comply with established standards of professional practice, hospital and departmental policies and procedures and identify impediments to optimal staff performance

- Define efficiency levels for various sections, functions and individual staff members within the department, determine whether preestablished levels of efficiency are being met and identify activities that improve or enhance the efficiency of the department and staff

- Appraise staffing needs and devise the most appropriate plan for assigning staff

- Anticipate the need for equipment, supplies and other resources and determine what equipment, supplies and resources should be upgraded and/or redeployed to more efficiently meet demands for service

- Determine the degree of user satisfaction and the cause of user dissatisfaction with departmental services

- Assess the safety of the environment

- Review the effect of nursing care on patient outcomes for specific patient groups or for patients with certain nursing diagnoses

- Identify episodes and problems which may expose the hospital or the department and its staff to liability

- Comply with JCAH, AOA and regulatory agencies' standards for QA data collection and evaluation

- Determine collaboratively with other disciplines or departments the effects their performance has on the operations of the nursing department

After defining the purposes of data collection, nurse managers must then establish a program for gathering the data on a timely and organized basis. A comprehensive and systematic monitoring program, if well planned, can do just that. However, to establish a successful monitoring program, managers must first understand the concept and structure of a monitor.

What Is a Monitor?

The hospital literature abounds with narrow definitions of monitoring. Monitoring has been defined solely as the means for meeting JCAH and regulatory agencies' requirements or as a method for uncovering any potential exposure to legal claims. However, because of the growing demands on nurse managers to develop and maintain a monitoring system that addresses quality, utilization, costs, compliance with standards, productivity, user satisfaction and exposure to risk, a monitor must have a broad definition. In this book, a monitor is defined as

> *a mechanism for repeatedly measuring and evaluating*
> *various aspects of hospital and departmental performance*

Unlike other hospital literature, this is not a monitoring "cookbook" with preselected criteria to be reviewed ad infinitum. In this book, we carefully refine monitors.

We DO present	**We DO NOT present**
A system for planning and implementing a comprehensive monitoring program that will meet the individual needs of nurse managers	Examples that a nurse manager must live with whether or not they apply to his/her department
Examples and suggestions that were drawn from interviews and working sessions with nurse managers and clinical nurse specialists in many hospitals	Theoretical examples that reflect superficial knowledge of the real problems faced by nurse and hospital managers
A review of the current professional literature specific to nursing	

We also show how to prepare an Agenda of Department Monitors that will guide the initial monitoring program and trace changes in the program

The Importance of Establishing an Agenda of Department Monitors

Since nursing is such a widespread and diverse service in hospitals, the number and scope of available monitors are perhaps the greatest of any of the inpatient departments. Because of the large number and wide variety of monitors, monitoring efforts in nursing are often impractical. Energy becomes so dispersed that the identification and resolution of important clinical problems is slow or completely lost in day-to-day operational activities. The importance of careful assessment and planning for meaningful monitors cannot be overemphasized.

Managers in nursing services and their staff, therefore, must make choices "upfront" about what realistically can be achieved through monitoring and prepare an Agenda to help them document the selection process and determine the types of resources that must be allocated and requested. A formal monitoring Agenda allows managers in nursing services to choose monitors that will make the best use of resources and yield the greatest payoff in useful information.

Although some regulations require certain types of monitors to be conducted on a continuous basis, the selection of most monitors is left to the discretion of nurse managers and their staff. Many managers do not wish to tie themselves and their departments to an ironclad list of "forever" monitors; so they are developing a year-to-year monitoring strategy. They will continuously (daily/weekly/monthly/ from year to year) conduct some monitors but will conduct other monitors only intermittently or for a limited period of time. With an Agenda, managers in nursing services can keep track of all these monitors.

An Agenda also can help managers identify new concerns that may require special monitoring or old monitors that are no longer fruitful and to establish and update monitoring priorities.

Overview Of The Contents Of The Monitoring Sourcebook

The nursing department offers a range of general and specialty services. This comprehensive resource on monitoring the variety of nursing services may be overwhelming if one tries to master all aspects of the proposed system in a short period of time. Therefore, readers will need to study and discuss each step in the monitoring process to fully understand how to best adapt it to their institution.

Because this book has been designed specifically for managers in nursing services, it identifies the topics, the data to be collected and the criteria that can be used for evaluating information in that department. Certain suggested topics and strategies for monitoring may not be feasible for some institutions at this time because the information systems needed to collect the data are not yet available. However, they are included to meet the future needs of nurse managers.

CHAPTER 2 presents certain perspectives about monitoring, including monitoring as a collaborative venture, monitoring and the JCAH and monitoring and the use of computers.

CHAPTER 3 breaks a monitor down into its component parts.

CHAPTER 4 presents a step-by-step approach for selecting monitoring topics. The approach includes review of the seven categories of monitors that are most commonly included in a departmental monitoring program.

CHAPTER 5 offers suggestions on how to integrate the monitoring effort into the day-by-day operation of the nursing department. Advice is given on what activities should be decentralized so all professional staff have accountability in the program.

CHAPTER 6 presents an extensive list of Department-specific topics under the seven major categories of monitors that are applicable to a variety of clinical nursing areas. These topics are used throughout the book as examples to illustrate the many technical points presented. The chapter also introduces the Unit/Department Monitoring Profile, a form that can be used to evaluate the department's current monitoring program and select high-priority topics.

CHAPTER 7 describes how to evaluate the appropriateness of current monitoring efforts and how to select high priority monitors.

CHAPTER 8 illustrates how to complete an Agenda of Department Monitors so data can be collected and results can be analyzed. The chapter outlines how to specify for each monitoring topic:

- Data to be collected

- Data sources

- Frequency and amount of data collection

- Content and frequency of summary data

- Duration of monitor

- Person to collect and summarize data

- Criteria for evaluating summary data and initiating further investigation

- Criteria sources

CHAPTER 9 shows examples of Agendas of Department Monitors with complete specifications for department-specific monitoring topics.

CHAPTER 10 provides a list of specific topics under the seven major categories of monitors for the following specialty clinical areas:

- Special care

- Maternal/child health

- Psychiatry/mental health

- Emergency department

- Operating room/recovery room

Although monitoring can help managers discover and correct problems in the efficiency and quality of services, a monitoring program cannot be effective unless it is done systematically. The purpose of this book is to guide the manager in nursing services in the preparation of a monitoring program that will yield information he/she can use to make sound management decisions and to improve the quality of services. Such a monitoring program will benefit the department, the hospital, the professional staff and the patients they serve.

2: Perspectives on Monitoring

Monitoring As A Collaborative Venture

In the planning of any monitoring program, the department manager plays the most significant role. Department managers are not totally on their own, however. In fact, our research has revealed that a successful departmental monitoring program is now a thoroughly collaborative effort.

Since the nursing services department affects and is affected by virtually all other departments that provide care to patients, the need for cooperation is imperative. Without cooperation from outside professionals, nurse managers may not be able to obtain the data they need to institute specific monitors in the most efficient manner.

For examples nurse managers may consult

- Quality assurance (QA), utilization review (UR), risk management (RM), safety, medical records, financial/billing and management engineering professionals to help select topics for monitoring, set specifications for monitors, collect data and provide pertinent reports to the department.

- Data-base coordinators and data-processing professionals to help set up systems to collect, store and retrieve data, perform calculations to be included in summary reports and produce and provide summary data reports specified by a monitor

- Clinical and administrative committees to help suggest topics for monitors, request summary data reports and use data generated by monitors to solve problems that involve clinicians and staff outside the department

The monitoring process described in this volume takes these types of collaboration into full account.

In addition to collaboration with other departments that can provide data **to** nursing, nursing evaluators find that they are increasingly called on to work **with** other clinical departments to monitor the:

- Clinical appropriateness of orders based on the patient's needs, symptoms and history and the results of testing

- Appropriateness of response to assessments, test results and recommendations

Monitoring As A Requirement Of The JCAH

One of the principal reasons for maintaining a departmental monitoring program is to meet the JCAH's QA requirements. Although the language in the QA standards has changed and the standards themselves have been interpreted inconsistently throughout the years, one aspect of the QA standards has remained constant: Hospital departments should collect information on the performance of the functions that affect patient care and should use that information to improve patient care whenever possible. To reinforce the concept of planned, formal QA data collection, JCAH standards now include a requirement for *MONITORING*. The QA standards are now stated uniformly for each department:

A. The nursing department/service has a planned and systematic process for the monitoring and evaluation of the quality and appropriateness of patient care and for resolving identified problems.

   1. The nurse administrator is responsible for assuring that the process is implemented.

B. The quality and appropriateness of patient care are monitored and evaluated in all major clinical functions of the nursing department/service. Such monitoring and evaluation are accomplished through the following means:

   1. Routine collection in the nursing department/service, or through the hospital quality assurance program, of information about important aspects of nursing care; and

   2. Periodic assessment by the nursing department/service of the collected information in order to identify important problems in patient care services and opportunities to improve care.

      a) In B.1 and B.2, the nursing department/service agrees on objective criteria that reflect current knowledge and clinical experience.

         (1) These criteria are used by the nursing department/service or by the hospital's quality assurance program in the monitoring and evaluation of patient care services.[1]

---

[1] Joint Commission on Accreditation of Hospitals: *Accreditation Manual for Hospitals,* 1987.

What constitutes an acceptable departmental monitor or an acceptable monitoring effort is not spelled out in these standards. The choices of monitoring topics, sources of data and criteria are appropriately left to the discretion of hospital professionals. Many hospital managers therefore are not sure whether their monitoring effort *will* conform to the JCAH surveyors' idea of "acceptable" monitoring. Managers are concerned that surveyors will not consider certain topics "relevant" or the scope of the monitoring program sufficient. Managers worry that certain utilization, productivity, safety or quality control monitors "won't count" because they are not "clinical" enough.

A monitoring program in nursing will **not** meet JCAH QA standards if it only includes monitors of utilization, charges and costs (eg, percent of time spent in non-patient care activities or costs of nursing care per diagnosis-related group [DRG]); standard quality control activities (eg, equipment checks or crash cart checks) and productivity measurement, (eg, average nursing care hours per DRG or the number of patients treated per shift, day or month in each patient acuity level). Nor will the monitoring program meet JCAH requirements if it collects only data about the number of nursing procedures performed (eg, number of IV starts, number of resuscitations).

The nursing QA program should be extended to address the appropriateness of decision making by nurses, appropriateness of performance by nurses of clinical procedures and the effect of nursing interventions on patients' outcomes (eg, was the appropriate technique followed in starting the IV? were complications avoided? were resuscitations successful? was the patient's status several hours following the resuscitation appropriate based on his pre-code condition?)

Nursing evaluators can gain additional insight by learning what accreditation surveyors themselves look for as they determine the adequacy of the QA effort in nursing.

Accreditation surveyors check on **what** is being evaluated.

1. Is the data generated by evaluation activities fully representative of nursing services provided to patients in the institution? Does the data cover:

    - The most common diagnostic and therapeutic procedures performed?

    - The services provided on all units and services of the institution?

    - The practice of all professionals who provide such services?

    - All the steps involved in the delivery of nursing services and in the clinical management of patients who receive these services?

2. As necessary, does the data generated through the evaluation effort focus on those procedures, types of cases or aspects of clinical management that are deemed or proven to be most problematic (ie, those that pose the highest risk to patients; those that produce the highest number of adverse outcomes, complications or injuries; those for which skills are likely to differ between new and experienced nurses; those that are the most overutilized/underutilized)?

3. Is data being generated on such "clinical" aspects of nursing care as:

    - The appropriateness of nursing assessments

    - The appropriateness of orders for nursing services?

- The competence of the staff who deliver services?

- The nature of the patient's response to the interventions that have been provided?

Surveyors are concerned about how the evaluation is designed and conducted.

1. Is data collection timely and contemporaneous with the care that is provided?

2. Is data collection sufficient to draw reasonable conclusions and to detect and identify problems or opportunities to improve care?

3. Are defensible criteria used in the evaluation?

4. Is the data summarized and reviewed with sufficient frequency?

5. Are appropriate management and clinical staff involved in the review of the data?

6. Is the evaluation data compared against appropriate and realistic goals?

JCAH surveyors consider followup to be the most important aspect of the evaluation process. They consequently assess whether the results of evaluation activities are acted upon in a timely and realistic manner.

1. Are problematic results of evaluation dealt with as quickly as possible by those with the authority and responsibility to do so?

2. What is the impact of the actions that were taken in response to evaluation results?

3. Does followup data demonstrate that the problems or issues identified through evaluation have been resolved?

Surveyors closely scrutinize actions. Often they will use available documentation to "track" problems, attempting to determine if staff was made accountable for the resolution of clinical practice problems. Surveyors expect the nurse managers to do more than just deliberate periodic monitoring results or communicate their concerns to one or more members of the nursing staff. Increasingly, they are looking for interventions aimed at changing clinical procedures and protocols, or altering the practice of individual clinicians. Finally, the JCAH representatives expect to see a formal linkage between evaluation results and the performance appraisals of individual staff members.

External Quality Reviews

Although they greatly influence the scope and direction of the QA evaluation effort in nursing, JCAH standards are not the "only game in town." State and federal requirements for assessing the quality of care delivered to enrollees in publicly financed health insurance programs, such as Medicare and Medicaid, also need to be heeded.

State and federal agencies are mandating that designated review groups, such as peer review organizations (PROs), identify clients of publicly financed health programs who may have received substandard or inappropriate care. More than likely, the entire continuum of the clinical management of patients will become a major focus of these evaluations as governmental agencies seek data to judge whether patients:

- Were initially placed at the appropriate level of care, consistent with the severity of their illness

- Were assessed and received necessary care in a manner that was timely and appropriate to the severity and nature of their condition

- Achieved acceptable outcomes prior to discharge or transfer to a less intensive care setting

- Were appropriately referred for continued aftercare

- Experienced serious adverse outcomes or complications that could have been avoided

Unlike the results of evaluations conducted for the JCAH, findings from "quality reviews" conducted by federal and state agencies will be made public. It therefore behooves nursing evaluators to have in place an evaluation mechanism that will anticipate and respond to data generated by outside reviewers.

The next chapters present a system for selecting monitors, six categories of monitors and department-specific examples for each category. The categories comprise a comprehensive monitoring program that will conform to the language and intent of JCAH standards.

Monitoring And Computers

Most nursing managers agree that a comprehensive monitoring program is an important though time-consuming and costly undertaking. For even if nurse managers are extremely selective in their choice of monitors, they and their staff will spend many hours collecting and analyzing data, and many nurse managers may find it difficult to believe that QA activities take up too many departmental resources and interfere with the efficient delivery of patient care services. Although hospital QA/UR professionals can provide some support and guidance, the department must use its own technical expertise and professional experience to conduct monitors.

The installation and enhancement of hospital and department computer-based information systems has offered a partial answer to the data collection problem. Although computer-based data sets are providing increasingly sophisticated, convenient and comprehensive information for nurse managers and other professionals, they are not an instantaneous source of information for all monitoring efforts, and trying to adapt these systems to handle departmental monitoring can be difficult.

Nurse managers must, for example, contend with these problems:

- Departmental and hospital automated information systems are often incompatible. Their hardware and software systems often do not "talk" to one another.

- The current systems are primarily used to generate data on utilization of departmental services and rough estimates of the costs and profitability of various services. Some systems are programmed to generate data on the timeliness of service, workflow, workload and productivity of staff. The systems do not usually, however, store data that can be used to evaluate the appropriateness of utilization or the quality of staff performance.

- In many hospitals, there are as yet no formal procedures to guide the access to, screening or distribution of data from hospital-wide information systems. And in the absence of formal procedures to guide their generation and use, hospital computer reports can become an undifferentiated mass of paper.

- Nurse managers often are not given the chance to recommend the data items that should be maintained in and generated by the hospital-wide computer system for purposes of QA monitoring.

- Nurse managers and staff usually do not have extensive knowledge of or experience with automated data bases and information systems. Without a sufficient understanding of the capabilities as well as the limitations of computers and information systems, nurse managers may have unrealistic expectations of the types of outputs that can be produced by these systems, or they may misuse the outputs in making important decisions.

  Although managers in all areas of nursing services must become educated about computer technology, they must remember that computers are only tools. Computers quickly assimilate, organize and display quantifiable data, but it is the manager who must judge the applicability and importance of the data to make sound decisions. Computer systems can *support* managers' decisions; they *cannot dictate* those decisions.

Computerization is revolutionizing the collection of information in hospitals, and it will continue to do so in the future. The full promise of computerization has not been realized, however. To be effective, hospital information systems probably will have to undergo a lengthy period of evolution. In the meantime, managers in nursing services must learn what is and is not available in the hospital information system so they can decide how the system can be used in monitoring. In addition, those who are responsible for maintaining the hospital information system must learn what kind of information nurse managers need for monitoring.

3. The Structure of a Monitor

As a mechanism for repeated measurement and evaluation, a monitor must have the following components: a topic, the type and sources of data to collect on that topic, the details regarding the frequency and duration of data collection, the person who will collect the data and criteria against which data will be compared.

Topic

The **Topic of a Monitor** is the function, service, procedure, section, shift, professional staff member or group, piece of equipment, type of supplies and/or patient group that will be assessed. Topics of monitors fall into seven broad categories:

Category I.   Utilization Monitors

Measure the demand for and use of departmental services by physicians, nurses and patients as well as by individuals from other disciplines, departments and services.

Category II.   Departmental Performance Monitors

Measure the quality and efficiency of performance by nurses of the nursing process in the care of patients and the impact of nursing intervention on patient outcomes.

Category III.   User Satisfaction Monitors

Measure the perceptions of the adequacy of departmental services held by physicians, patients, patient family members and hospital staff.

Category IV.   Safety Monitors

Review the environment in which departmental procedures are performed, the potential and known hazards to patients and staff and the readiness of staff to recognize and respond to hazards.

Category V.   Quality Control Monitors

Review the attainment and maintenance of expected credentialing and skill levels by departmental personnel. They also review the quality of equipment and supplies used in the course of providing services.

Category VI.   Incident/Occurrence Monitors

Review episodes of actual or potential patient or employee harm.

Category VII.   Monitors of Patient Management and Clinical Practices of Other Departments

Measure the practices and performance of staff from other departments that affect the daily operations of nursing services.

For purposes of illustration, this chapter will use the following topic examples:

Category I.   Utilization: Appropriateness of admissions to general care units according to nursing staffing patterns

Category II.   Departmental Performance: Adherence to protocols for maintaining patients on total parenteral nutrition (TPN)

Category III.   User Satisfaction: Patient satisfaction with the clarity and completeness of the written discharge instructions given by nursing personnel

Category IV.   Safety: Compliance of unit personnel to the procedure for reporting and responding to fire drills on the unit

Category V.   Quality Control: Integrity/readiness of the unit crash cart for responding to CPR codes

Category VI.   Incident/Occurrence: Unintended outcomes following tube feedings administered to patients by nursing personnel. (eg, diarrhea, aspiration pneumonia, administration of feeding into lungs due to tube displacement)

Category VII.   Patient Management and Clinical Practices of Other Departments: Appropriateness/accuracy of monitoring patients' IV infusions by radiology technologists when patients are in the radiology department for treatment or tests

Data

Data to be Collected for a monitor details the precise events, items and variables that should be counted or measured and/or the criteria that should be applied.

Data Sources specify the best sources—either inside or outside the department—for obtaining information about the events, items and/or variables that must be collected.

Examples

Category I: Utilization

Topic: Appropriateness of admissions to general care units according to nursing staffing patterns

    Data to be collected:

- Number of admissions of patients by
  - patient diagnosis
  - type of admission (eg, emergency, urgent, elective, etc)
  - condition of patient (if critical, serious or fair)
  - assigned unit
  - shift during which patient was admitted to the unit
- Number and mix of nursing personnel on each unit during each shift
- Number of patient care hours required for each unit at the beginning of each shift

    Data sources: Admission, discharge and transfer (ADT) computer file, staffing/scheduling log, acuity reports for each shift on the general care units

Category II: Departmental Performance

Topic: Adherence to protocols for maintaining patients on TPN

    Data to be collected:

- Number of patients receiving TPN
- Number of cases with deviations from protocols
- Number and type of deviations from protocols (by type of deviation), including absence of
  - documentation of vital signs, Clinitest results, daily weights, tubing changes, dressing changes, I&O measurements
  - IV infusion pump for administering solution
  - tubing with appropriate filter
  - labels on tubing and/or dressing
  - administration of other medications via the TPN line
- Number of nurses who have been observed completing the central line dressing changes
- Number of deviations from dressing change procedure (by nurse and type of deviation)
- Number of patients with infection associated with TPN

    Data sources: Patients' medical records, clinical unit's IV therapy log, observation of nurses during nursing grand rounds using a prepared checklist, observation of nurses by peers and the unit nurse educator using a checklist of departmental policies and procedures, interview with the infection control nurse

Category III: User Satisfaction

Topic: Patient satisfaction with the clarity and completeness of the written discharge instructions given by nursing personnel

Data to be collected: Patient responses to the following questions

1. Did you receive a copy of the discharge instructions form?
2. Was it legible?
3. Could you understand all the information and terms?
4. Did the discharge information form have all the information you needed to continue your therapy at home? If not, what instructions should have been included?
5. Have you been able to follow all the instructions about your therapy since your discharge from the hospital? If not, what instructions would have enabled you to continue your therapy at home?

Data source: Telephone interviews, copies of the discharge instruction forms

Category IV: Safety

Topic: Compliance of unit personnel to the procedure for reporting and responding to fire drills on the unit

Data to be collected: For each shift and unit

- Actions (in sequence) taken by the person or persons who discover the "fire"
- Deviations from the standard procedure for responding to a fire, such as
  -closing all doors and windows
  -moving patients away from the "fire" (if necessary)
  -shutting off oxygen
  -preparing charts for removal from the unit
- Type of personnel responsible for deviations from procedure

Data source: Observation using a checklist of departmental policies and procedures

Category V: Quality Control

Topic: Integrity/readiness of the unit crash cart for responding to CPR codes

Data to be collected: Answers to the following questions

- Is the crash cart secured/locked?
- Is the crash cart in the proper location?
- Are all designated pieces of equipment on the crash cart?
- Are all designated pieces of equipment in working order?

- Are all designated medications on the crash cart?
- Are doses of designated medications correct? Are any medications outdated?

Data source: Crash cart checklist

Category VI: Incident/Occurrence

Topic: Unintended outcomes following tube feedings administered to patients by nursing personnel (eg, diarrhea, aspiration pneumonia, administration of feeding into lungs due to tube displacement)

Data to be collected: For every shift and unit
- Number of patients receiving tube feedings
- Number and type of unintended adverse outcome
- Patient ID number
- Patient diagnosis
- Patient age
- Patient care unit on which adverse outcome occurred

Data sources: Incident reports, medical record abstracts and log kept by nursing personnel

Category VII: Patient Management and Clinical Practices of Other Departments:

Topic: Appropriateness/accuracy of monitoring patients' IV infusions by radiology technologists when patients are in the radiology department for treatment or tests

Data to be collected:
- Number of incidents of inadequate monitoring, including
  -incorrect IV solution given
  -incorrect rate of infusion
  -dislodged needle
  -clotted needle
  -IV "running dry"
- Scores for each radiology technologist on pre- and post-tests of the following tasks
  -evaluation of the IV site for infiltration
  -maintenance of a patient on IV (eg, preventing clot formation in the needle, changing solutions, preventing IVs from "running dry")
  -evaluation of IV rate
  -timely checks of the IV (eg, after any repositioning or transfer of the patient)

Data sources: Log kept by the nursing staff and radiology supervisor, pre- and post-test questionnaires

Frequency and Duration of Data Collection

The Frequency and Amount of Data Collection specifies the amount of data that will be collected on each event, item and/or variable and how frequently data will be collected.

Content and Frequency of Summary Reports itemizes the statistics that should be compiled, calculated and reported and how frequently the statistics should be reported.

The Duration of the Monitor specifies when monitors should begin (start) and end (stop) and when they should be reappraised to determine if the data should be modified or if the monitor should be discontinued completely.

Examples

Category I: Utilization

Topic: Appropriateness of admissions to general care units according to nursing staffing patterns

Frequency and amount of data collection: Admissions during 21 sequential shifts should be reviewed.

Content and frequency of summary reports: The following report will be submitted to the nursing management committee each month, and data will be summarized quarterly:

- Total number of admissions reviewed
- Frequency of admission to each shift and unit that have the following Productivity Indices. (In this example, a Productivity Index is equal to the total number of patient care hours that are required divided by the number of nursing care hours that are available. For a more complete discussion of Productivity Indices, see page 49.)
  Productivity Index = 90% or lower
  Productivity Index = 91-94%
  Productivity Index = 95-99%
  Productivity Index = 100% or above
- Number of times patients were admitted to a unit with a Productivity Index of 100% or above when a unit with an index of 90% or below was available. (Specify the unit and the shift.)
- Number of times a patient classified as critical, serious or fair was assigned to a unit with a Productivity Index of 95% or above. (Specify the unit and shift.)

Duration of Monitor: October and June; reappraise in June

Category II: Departmental Performance

Topic: Adherence to protocols for maintaining patients on TPN

*Frequency and amount
of data collection:*   Review all cases one day a week for eight weeks. Then review all cases one day a month for three months.

*Content and frequency
of summary reports:*   The following report will be submitted to the nursing QA committee monthly for the first eight weeks of the monitoring period and then quarterly for the next three months.

- Total number of cases reviewed

- Total number and percent distribution of discrepancies from protocols (by type of discrepancy)

- Number of nurses observed changing dressings

- Number and type of deviations from procedures for changing dressings (by nurse)

- Infection rate related to TPN

Monthly summaries of the observation of nurses on each unit will be given to the head nurse of the unit.

Duration: June to October

Category III: User Satisfaction

Topic: Patient satisfaction with the clarity and completeness of the written discharge instructions given by nursing personnel

*Frequency and amount
of data collection:*   A total of 15 patients should be randomly selected from each month's discharges and interviewed monthly.

*Content and frequency
of summary reports:*   Reports of the frequency of the responses to each question and the patients' comments should be prepared monthly and summarized quarterly. The reports should be submitted to the professional practice committee in the nursing department and the nursing QA committee.

Duration: From March to May and for another quarter after changes based on patient responses have been made.

Category IV: Safety

Topic: Compliance of unit personnel to the procedure for reporting and responding to fire drills on the unit

Frequency and amount of data collection: Information on each shift should be collected every six months.

Content and frequency of summary reports: The number and types of deviations from established procedures should be reported by shift, by unit and for all shifts and units. Reports should be prepared semiannually and submitted to the nursing QA committee and the hospital safety committee.

Duration: Continuous

Category V: Quality Control

Topic: Integrity/readiness of the unit crash carts for responding to CPR codes

Frequency and amount of data collection: Integrity of the lock on the crash cart should be checked during each shift; the presence and functional use of designated equipment and medications should be checked weekly and after each use.

Content and frequency of summary reports: Reports of the frequency of each type of deviation should be prepared monthly for each unit. A report of the frequency of each deviation should be submitted to the nursing QA committee, quarterly.

Duration: Continuous

Category VI: Incident/Occurrence

Topic: Unintended outcomes following tube feedings administered to patients by nursing personnel (such as, diarrhea, aspiration pneumonia, administration of feeding into lungs due to tube displacement)

Frequency and amount of data collection: Information should be collected on all unintended outcomes on every shift and on every unit.

Content and frequency of summary reports: The following report should be prepared monthly for the nursing QA committee and the RM committee.

- Total number of unintended outcomes for the entire nursing services department and for each patient care unit
- Total number of each type of unintended outcome for the entire nursing services department and for each patient care unit

A monthly report of the total number of unintended outcomes and the number of each type of outcome on each unit should be given to the head nurse of the unit.

Duration: From January to June; reappraise in June

Category VII: Patient Management and Clinical Practices of Other Departments

Topic: Appropriateness/accuracy of monitoring patients' IV infusions by radiology technologists when patients are in the radiology department for treatments or tests

Frequency and amount of data collection: All lapses of IV monitoring should be reviewed during one quarter. Data from a pre- and post-test questionnaire for radiology technologists should be collected and summarized.

Content and frequency of summary reports: The following report will be prepared jointly by nursing and radiology and presented to the hospital QA committee quarterly.

- Total number of incidents logged
- Frequency and percent distribution of incidents (by type)
- Total number of questionnaires completed by radiology technologists
- Total number (percent) of correct responses to questions
- Frequency and percent distribution of correct responses for each question

Duration of monitor: October to December to determine the extent of the problem, March to June following the implementation of a training program for radiology technologists (if needed)

Person/Criteria

Person to Collect and Summarize Data identifies the staff members from inside and outside the department who will collect and summarize the data for the monitor.

Criteria to Evaluate Summary Data and Initiate Further Investigation specifies the desired level of achievement or goal against which the summary data will be compared, indicates when the goal was not attained, and points to the need for the department manager to investigate the potential problem. Some monitors do not require criteria (eg, monitors that seek suggestions and comments for improving departmental operations, that compare the quality, cost and efficiency of different treatment modalities or pieces of equipment or that collect baseline information on the utilization of services and cost of running the department).

Criteria Sources indicate where a department manager can search for recognized levels of achievement for each monitor, including hospital and departmental policies and procedures, job descriptions, standards established by professional associations or reported in the professional literature and the manager's own education and experience.

Examples:

Category I: Utilization

Topic: Appropriateness of admissions to general care units according to nursing staffing patterns

Persons to collect and summarize data: A committee will be formed and will include a nurse liaison in the admitting department, a coordinator for nursing resources and one manager and one staff nurse from general units.

Criteria to evaluate summary data and initiate further investigation: Any of the following situations will result in further investigation.

- A patient was assigned to a unit whose Productivity Index was 100% or above when another unit had an index of 90% or below.
- A patient classified as critical, serious or fair was admitted to a unit whose Productivity Index was 95% or greater.
- A patient was assigned to a unit whose Productivity Index was 100% or greater for 20% or more shifts during the monitoring period.

During the second quarter of monitoring, the following must be met.

- Assignment of patients to a unit whose Productivity Index is 100% or above will not exceed a rate of 20% for all shifts.
- Assignment of patients to units with a Productivity Index of 100% or above when other units have an index of 90% or below will be reduced to zero.
- Assignment of patients classified as critical, serious or fair to units with a Productivity Index of 95% or above will be reduced to zero.

Criteria sources: Professional judgment of executive committee of nurse managers

Category II: Departmental Performance

Topic: Adherence to protocols for maintaining patients on TPN

Persons to collect and summarize data: An ad hoc nursing committee will collect and summarize data.

Criteria to evaluate summary data and initiate further investigation:
- Adherence to protocols for maintaining patients on TPN should be 100%.

- Adherence to procedures for changing dressings should be 100%.
- The infection rate associated with TPN should be no more than 3% by the end of the next two quarters.

Failure to meet these criteria will result in the creation of an institutional credentialing procedure for nurses who are responsible for monitoring TPN.

Criteria sources: Professional literature, departmental policies and procedures

Category III: User Satisfaction

Topic: Patient satisfaction with the clarity and completeness of the written discharge instructions given by nursing personnel

Person to collect
and summarize data: A member of the nursing QA committee and a volunteer staff nurse should work together each month to collect and summarize the data.

Criteria to evaluate
summary data and initiate
further investigation: The rate of positive responses should be at least 95% for each individual item and for all items combined after the first quarter of the monitor and 99% after the second quarter of the monitor. Failure to meet these goals will result in action by the nursing QA committee in conjunction with the Nurse Management Forum.

Any patient comment that suggests the possibility of litigation will be followed up individually by the hospital ombudsman.

Criteria sources: Professional judgment

Category IV: Safety

Topic: Compliance of unit personnel to the procedure for reporting and responding to fire drills on the unit

Person to collect
and summarize data: The unit nurse manager or assistant should collect data and a member of the safety committee should summarize them.

Criteria to evaluate
summary data and initiate
further investigation: There should be 100% compliance to departmental policies and procedures.

Criteria source: Nursing departmental policies and procedures

Category V: Quality Control
Topic: Integrity/readiness of the unit crash cart for responding to CPR codes

*Person to collect
and summarize data:*   Charge nurse on each shift should collect data and pharmacy supervisor should summarize them.

*Criteria to evaluate
summary data and initiate
further investigation:*   The integrity/readiness of the crash cart must be maintained 100% of the time. Any inadequacies will be investigated and corrected immediately.

Criteria sources: Regulations of the state department of health and the JCAH. Pharmacy and nursing departments' policies and procedures.

Category VI: Incident/Occurrence
Topic: Unintended outcomes following feedings administered to patients by nursing personnel (eg, diarrhea, aspiration pneumonia, administration of feeding into lungs due to tube displacement)

*Person to collect
and summarize data:*   The hospital risk manager and the medical-surgical clinical nurse specialist should work together to summarize the data collected by a staff nurse volunteer on each unit.

*Criteria to evaluate
summary data and initiate
further investigation:*   Any unintended outcome that appears each month on any one unit or whose total monthly frequency is greater than one percent will be investigated.

Criteria sources: Professional judgment of the nursing QA committee and the hospital risk manager

Category VII: Patient Management and Clinical Practices of Other Departments
Topic: Appropriateness/accuracy of monitoring patients' IV infusions by radiology techs when patients are in the radiology department for treatments or tests

*Person to collect
and summarize data:*   A task force will be created by the hospital QA committee and will include representatives from the nursing services and radiology departments and the risk manager for the hospital

*Criteria to evaluate
summary data and initiate
further investigation:*   The number of incidents of inadequate IV monitoring by radiology technologists will be reduced by 90% by the end of the second quarter of monitoring. All technologists must achieve 100% correct responses on the post-test questionnaire.

Criteria sources: Policies of the radiology department and job descriptions of radiology technologists

More detailed directions for completing the specifications for a monitor are presented in Chapter 8.

4: Types and Categories of Monitors

Types of Monitors

Before nurse managers try to establish a comprehensive departmental monitoring system, they may find it helpful to review the major types of monitors that are used in other departments and hospitals. A preliminary assessment of these monitors allows nurse managers to define the scope of their monitoring program, to evaluate current monitoring activities and to plan changes in these activities.

In a comprehensive monitoring effort, there are two basic types of monitors.

Type 1: Scanning Monitors

provide general data about the functioning or performance of a department or the utilization of its services. Most often, SCANNING MONITORS are used to generate critical statistics about overall operations. With SCANNING MONITORS, managers select the variables that will provide the best overview of the departmental functioning.

Nurse managers who make use of SCANNING MONITORS may choose such variables as:

- Ratio of nursing care hours required to nursing care hours provided (productivity index)

- Number of codes for CPR and survival rate by unit

- Average performance score on CPR drills for all clinical units and shifts

- Rate of incidents reported by type of incident for the department and each unit (eg, medication errors, falls, etc)

- Rate of nosocomial infections for the department and each unit

- Statistical distribution of patient falls according to the time of day, the patient's activity at the time of the fall, the use of siderails (if applicable), the use of restraints (if applicable)

- Statistical distribution of patients' acuity levels by DRG or unit

- Statistical distribution of emergency patients by acuity level, such as non-emergent, emergent, urgent and critical

- Statistical distribution of low-risk and high-risk mothers in obstetrical areas by physician and payor category

- Frequency with which nurses provide respiratory services to pediatric patients due to unavailability of respiratory therapy staff

- Average nursing care hours per patient for the 10 DRGs that have the highest estimated nursing costs

- Total number and percent of readmissions within 60 days of patients with diabetes mellitus

- Total number of nursing personnel in each service or unit who attend continuing education each quarter

- Total number and percent of urinary tract infections by unit for catherized patients

Once SCANNING MONITORS have been established, they often remain in place from year to year and summaries of their findings usually are prepared and reviewed at several preset times throughout the year. However, nurse managers should periodically review the usefulness of monitors for which data are collected manually and alter, delete or supplement the monitors as needed. Such continuous monitors are fine if the data is easily obtained (eg, from computerized printouts).

Examples

- A monitor in one institution for the number of codes for CPR on general clinical units indicated a steady increase in codes because criteria for admitting patients to special care units were too stringent. After the admitting criteria were revised, the nurse management group for special care units instituted a continuous SCANNING MONITOR of CPR codes on all general units. For each month over the next two quarters, the rate of codes for CPR was consistently below previous levels. Because of the life-threatening nature of the problem, the management group felt that CPR codes on general units should still be continuously monitored. However, since the rate of codes was dropping, the group decided to reduce the frequency of reporting data from monthly to quarterly.

- From a SCANNING MONITOR in one institution, nurse managers discovered many nursing personnel were signing to work open shifts on units other than their own. The overtime pay for the staff nurses involved was charged to their "home" unit making accurate budgeting for units impossible. Therefore, the nurse managers and support services personnel set up a procedure for tracking—and charging to the appropriate unit—the pay earned by staff nurses who worked shifts that had not been assigned by the scheduling office. Because subsequent monitoring indicated that overtime pay was reflected in the appropriate unit's budget, the nurse management group concluded that the immediate problem had been solved. While they saw no need to continuously monitor nurses' overtime, the group nonetheless felt that charges for overtime should be spotchecked periodically; so it scheduled a SCANNING MONITOR to run during two quarters each year.

- The nurse management group in one hospital anticipated that their case mix of patients would change as a result of prospective pricing systems. Therefore, they began to monitor the distribution of the patient population by DRG at departmental and unit levels. After reviewing monthly reports generated by the hospital's information system for two quarters, the group found that the data on patient population in all DRGs were too global. The group therefore replaced the SCANNING MONITOR of patients in all DRGs with one that gathered data on patients in the ten DRGs having the highest volume for the institution and the three DRGs having the highest volume for each clinical unit.

The statistics generated by means of a SCANNING MONITOR may be evaluated against a predetermined goal or standard. These goals or standards may be set internally or derived from comparative statistics, and they may describe:

- A threshold level that indicates when performance is substandard and action must be taken

- An ideal level that indicates optimal performance

- The degree of change that is desired

Examples

- *Topic:* Timeliness of written nursing care plan

  A quality assurance committee in nursing, with input from nurse managers and staff nurses, set 90 percent as a threshold level for the completion of nursing care plans on the medical record within 24 hours of admission.

- *Topic:* Nosocomial infections among patients

  An infection control committee, in collaboration with the nursing quality assurance committee, set 5 percent as a threshold level for the rate of nosocomial infections in the hospital.

- *Topic:* Timeliness of written admission assessments by nursing personnel

  The professional nurse practice committee established an ideal level of performance for completion of written nursing assessments. The committee stated that assessments by RNs should be done on all patients within the first full shift after admission.

- *Topic:*   Productivity of nursing personnel

  The executive nurse management group established for each clinical unit an ideal Productivity Index. The Productivity Index had an upper limit of 110 percent and a lower unit of 85 percent.

- *Topic:*   Accuracy of performance of CPR by direct care givers

  The risk management committee set 100 percent as an ideal yearly goal for CPR certification of direct patient care givers.

- *Topic:*   Falls of patients on clinical units

  A nursing department task force on patient falls expected a 25 percent change in the rate of falls after the institution of a "falls reduction program."

Whether or not they are evaluated against a preestablished goal, data generated through SCANNING MONITORS are often used to detect problems and raise concerns about the functioning of the department. However, since SCANNING MONITORS offer little detail, these monitors can only suggest the areas that require further investigation, a special study or a more focused monitoring effort.

Type 2:   Focused Monitors

provide continuous or intermittent information about (1) a specific function, section or procedure, (2) the utilization practices of a specific individual or group or (3) the services provided to a specific patient group. A FOCUSED MONITOR is needed when:

- The interdisciplinary team on an inpatient mental health unit is interested in determining whether eligible patients are receiving support services offered by the unit's clinical nurse specialist

- The nursing-pharmacy committee wishes to check on the turnaround time for administration of STAT medications that are not stock items on clinical units

- The nursing-dietetics committee wants to substantiate that all patients with a primary or secondary diagnosis of diabetes mellitus have a dietary evaluation within 48 hours of admission

The information generated from a FOCUSED MONITOR is used to determine the cause, nature or scope of a suspected or known problem in the functioning of the department or in the utilization of its services. The results of SCANNING MONITORS or other review activities often suggest the topics of FOCUSED MONITORS.

Examples

- After a SCANNING MONITOR disclosed an increasing rate of reported medication errors over one quarter, the nurse management group in one institution established a FOCUSED MONITOR to break down the overall error rate by unit and shift. The FOCUSED MONITOR uncovered a particularly high medication error rate during the night shift on four units. Further investigation revealed that these units had hired a number of new graduate nurses over the past quarter. At the same time, these units were caring for patients with high acuity levels. The nurse management group continued both the SCANNING and the FOCUSED MONITORS during the next six months while the nurse managers of the four units took remedial action. The group planned to discontinue the FOCUSED MONITOR, however, when the rate of medication errors fell to appropriate, preestablished levels.

- A SCANNING MONITOR of the incidence of decubitus ulcer formation during patients' hospital stay yielded a highly variable rate by unit. The quality assurance coordinator in nursing formed a task force, composed of staff members and managers from units whose rate of decubiti was 25 percent or more of the total number of hospital-acquired decubiti, to conduct a FOCUSED MONITOR of the clinical characteristics of patients who develop decubiti and the nursing care that is given before and after decubiti formation. The quality assurance coordinator hoped that the monitoring effort would define the patient population at risk of decubiti and indicate the preventive nursing measures that should be implemented. After specific preventive measures were instituted on these units, the quality assurance coordinator planned to establish another SCANNING MONITOR, which would continue on the targeted units until the number of decubiti decreased significantly.

The data generated by FOCUSED MONITORS are usually compared to preestablished goals or standards. The following goals/standards have been used in various hospitals.

- The nursing QA committee specified that there must be 100% compliance to the procedure for documenting the type and amount of intravenous (IV) solutions given a patient and the condition of the IV site.

- A task force monitoring the referral of specific patient populations to the nurse discharge planner felt that all patients with specific diagnoses should be referred within 24 hours of admission.

- When monitoring the use of float nurses as staff in critical care units, the critical care committee specified that all float personnel should be signed off on a list of specialized skills before being allowed to deliver care.

- The critical care committee at one hospital decided that each physician should meet 99 percent of the criteria for admitting and discharging patients to and from special care units.

The data generated from FOCUSED MONITORS are often used to plan or justify actions taken by managers or by administrative and clinical committees.

Examples

- A FOCUSED MONITOR of patients' satisfaction with instruction given by nurses on the care of a surgical wound indicated that teaching often was done too quickly almost immediately before discharge, with no opportunity for the patient or family member to demonstrate understanding of the instructions. This feedback led the nursing quality assurance committee to form a task force that would develop, implement and later evaluate a standard teaching program for surgical patients.

- By means of a FOCUSED MONITOR, the nurse manager of a cardiology unit noted that a number of patients with arrythmia were unstable intermittently during their length of stay. The data from this monitor helped the nurse manager justify the installation of telemetry on the unit.

- An orthopedic unit nurse manager believed the semi-private rooms were too small for acutely ill orthopedic patients to move about safely. She took pictures of a mock situation depicting patients' inability to maneuver in the bathroom or to ambulate with walkers and the staff's inability to reach patients if they fell in the bathroom. The nurse manager used a FOCUSED MONITOR to report the number of patients assigned to these rooms, the types of equipment and nursing care the patients needed and the potential injuries or untoward events that could occur because the rooms' size prevented staff from meeting patients' needs. The manager planned to use the data to demonstrate the need for converting a limited number of semiprivate rooms to private rooms and for remodeling the rooms to meet predetermined criteria.

FOCUSED MONITORS are time-limited; they generally are not carried over from year to year as SCANNING MONITORS are. Rather, they are discontinued once they substantiate that no real problem exists, reveal the nature and cause of a problem or demonstrate that a problem has been solved. Obviously, they may be reinstituted if a problem recurs.

Examples

- The nurse manager on a pediatric unit suspected that the professional nursing staff were spending too much time running off-unit errands to the pharmacy. She instituted a FOCUSED MONITOR to determine the exact amount of time professional staff members spent in this activity. After collecting data for one quarter, the monitor showed that the time nurses spent in off-unit errands to the pharmacy was not excessive; so the nurse manager discontinued the monitor.

- The majority of the medical staff in one institution ignored the discharge time of 11:30 a.m., causing an erratic daily flow of admissions to and discharges from nursing units. The staff and the nurse managers of medical/surgical units believed this practice decreased productivity of the day and afternoon nursing shifts, disrupted the assignment of patients to a primary nurse and delayed the initiation of therapeutic procedures for newly admitted patients. The nurse managers of the medical/surgical units instituted a FOCUSED MONITOR to determine the number of patients who stayed past 11:30 a.m. on their day of discharge, the exact time patients were discharged, the number of patients whose admission was delayed or whose placement in a unit was inappropriate because of the slow turnaround of beds and the number and nature of therapeutic procedures that were delayed because of the late admission of patients.

On the basis of the results of the monitor, the QA administrative committee, in conjunction with the medical staff, initiated a major educational program for attending physicians and house staff that reinforced the importance of adhering to the 11:30 a.m. discharge time. When a subsequent FOCUSED MONITOR indicated 50 percent improvement, the QA administrative committee discontinued the monitor. The committee did, however, request that the admissions/discharge office report to the QA coordinator whenever late discharges surpassed the current rate by 10 percent.

- Staff nurses from several clinical units reported to the nursing QA committee that laboratory test results were delayed because laboratory specimens were not drawn on time or because certain tests were run only at specific times of the day or week. The QA committee formed an interdepartmental ad hoc group, consisting of nursing and laboratory personnel, to monitor the problem and recommend solutions. The group collected data on the number and kinds of laboratory tests that were not done routinely on all shifts as well as the turnaround time from the physician's order for a lab test and the report of the test's results. The information yielded by the monitor led the laboratory manager to redistribute the staff's workload and change staffing patterns to obtain better coverage during "off-shifts." When subsequent monitoring indicated the problem had been resolved, the ad hoc group was disbanded, and the monitor was discontinued.

As indicated in examples under the different categories of monitors in this chapter and examples in subsequent chapters, many departmental monitoring programs have both SCANNING and FOCUSED monitors in progress.

Categories of Monitors

In addition to reviewing the types of monitors that other departments use, managers in nursing services also may find it helpful to learn how monitors can be classified according to the management and clinical information the monitors will generate. This review allows managers to precisely plan and systematically evaluate their monitoring programs.

Surveys and interviews conducted in many hospitals identified six major information categories of monitors for most departments and one category specific to nursing as well as a number of subgroups within these categories. In many hospitals nurse managers monitor topics in all these categories so they can amass a complete departmental data base.

> ### CATEGORY I. UTILIZATION MONITORS
>
> **Measure the demand for and use of nursing services by physicians, other nurses and patients as well as by individuals from other disciplines, departments and services.**

Data generated from Utilization Monitors can be used by nurse managers and administrators and clinical committees in the nursing department to:

- Estimate staffing, equipment and supply needs

- Detect and provide objective evidence of the appropriateness of demands for nursing services and thereby identify overutilization or underutilization of specific procedures and services

- Determine whether nursing care hours required by patients are met by the nursing care hours available for patient care

- Determine whether the results of patient assessments or professional recommendations made by nursing staff in the department are used appropriately by physicians, nurses and others in patient treatment decisions

Utilization Monitors in Nursing

In the initial phases of adapting to the prospective pricing system, hospital administrators have tended to focus on physicians' use of resources, particularly physicians' ordering patterns for ancillary services. Physicians have been asked to defend not only their decisions to admit patients but their diagnostic and therapeutic regimen after patients have been admitted and to justify their professional judgments by substantiating that their treatment decisions (1) have a positive impact on the quality of care, (2) decrease patients' length of stay and/or complication rates and (3) directly affect patient outcome.

Nurses must recognize that they will be asked to justify their professional judgments and activities in a similar way. Nurses cannot merely focus on what they "feel" is necessary to the delivery of appropriate nursing care in hospitals; they must prepare to defend their ordering practices with data that demonstrate the demand for nursing care time and other services is appropriate to the *current, documented* needs of the patient and result in (1) timely discharge of the patient, (2) lower complication rates and (3) improved standards of health care.

Staff nurses and nurse managers in the past have focused on the performance of nursing services; they often have *not* addressed the appropriateness of the *demand* for these services. Utilization Monitors obtain information on which this decision can be made. For example, monitors of physician- or nurse-ordering patterns for vital signs or intake and output levels may show that nurses continue to take these measurements whether or not the patients' condition warrants such extensive scrutiny.

Physical therapy, occupational therapy, respiratory therapy and other departments often expect nurses to continue their patient care functions during off-shifts, weekends or holidays. Utilization Monitors in nursing services can track and quantify such demands. The data from the monitors can be used to justify adjustments in the departmental budget for nursing or in staffing to accommodate the additional workload or to negotiate with the appropriate department over who should be responsible for performing these duties.

Utilization Monitors also can provide invaluable information on how staff nurses spend their time and help nurse managers decide how nurses' time *should* be spent.

Category I.   Utilization Monitors

Subcategory A.   Statistical Distribution of Orders, Referrals and Costs

Because of prospective pricing and capitation payment systems, hospitals must keep the costs of patient care within established reimbursement limits. Nursing services is usually the largest department in a health care institution, it accounts for a major part of the hospital's budget, and it performs a myriad of nursing and non-nursing services for patients. Yet the amount of information on the demands for services (in terms of orders/referrals for nursing care) and the costs that these demands incur is meager or nonexistent in many institutions.

Nurse managers may plan to collect statistical information on the overall orders and referrals or the orders/referrals for specific services over time. Managers may then use these statistics to indicate the distribution of demand by one or more preselected variables (eg, DRG, payor category, acuity level).

Although demands for nursing services are often described in hours of nursing care, the costs of nursing services traditionally have been part of the patients' room charge. Because of the prospective pricing system and the growth of the nursing profession itself, the federal government and individual hospitals are using other methods of costing out nursing services so that appropriate reimbursement and cost containment decisions can be made. This subcategory of Utilization Monitors can assist in these efforts by quantifying the demand for nursing care hours more specifically so the actual cost of nursing services for a single patient or groups of patients by diagnostic category can be determined.

Utilization by Diagnostic Group

Because the utilization of nursing services can determine whether a hospital makes a profit or suffers a loss for certain case-mix groups, hospital administrators need ongoing statistical information on the hours of nursing care spent in the treatment of patients in specific diagnostic groups. A variety of SCANNING and FOCUSED MONITORS are helping nurse managers focus their efforts on the case-mix groups and services that are most problematic for the nursing department and the institution as a whole. To generate useful data, such monitoring efforts require the close collaboration of nurse managers, staff nurses, clinical nurse specialists and professionals who maintain the hospital's case-mix accounting system. They also require a long-term commitment to a carefully thought-out plan. Instituting a series of case-mix group-related monitors may take months to unfold and to complete these preliminary steps:

- Establishing a reliable and valid patient classification acuity system that can capture the nursing care time needed by specific types of patients

- Establishing a mechanism by which the nursing acuity data from the patient classification system can be coupled with appropriate DRGs

- Computing nursing costs per DRG based on the nursing acuity system and the total cost of the nursing services department in the institution

- Accepting nurse managers' input into the hospital's case-mix system to ensure that data are correctly collected, coded and summarized in the overall case-mix data base

- Encouraging managers in nursing to meet with the individuals who oversee the hospital's case-mix accounting system in order to determine the types of reports that can be generated about departmental utlization and the reports that will be most helpful

- Restricting departmental managers', clinical committee members' and administrators' selection of variables that will be reported on each DRG, on the hundreds of separate categories of charges or on the practices of the entire medical staff. This step prevents the monitoring effort from becoming "choked" with printouts and masses of uninterpretable data.

Once these preliminary steps have been taken, nurse managers can begin to incorporate case-mix group-specific monitors into their overall monitoring program. To monitor the use of services by DRG in their departments, nurse managers may follow one of three strategies. These strategies are currently being used by managers in pharmacy, radiology and clinical laboratory to describe how managers can determine the use of services by DRG. As more refined case-mix or diagnostic data specific to nursing services become available, nurse managers can use these strategies as mechanisms for defining and interpreting the information they need and for determining the use of services for any diagnostic group selected by the hospital.

STRATEGY 1:   Monitoring the Nursing Department's Experience with the Hospital's "Top DRGs"

Managers who adopt this approach:

a. Identify the 10 or 20 DRGs that encompass the highest total number of patient admissions, patient days, charges or estimated costs for the hospital—or the 10 or 20 DRGs that account for the greatest net losses of revenue for the hospital.

b. Generate the following information for each "top DRG"

  - total dollar amount of departmental costs

  - percentage of total hospital charges/costs that were attributed to nursing services

  - average estimated departmental cost per patient

  - percentage of total departmental charges or estimated costs that were attributed to each DRG

c. Inititate departmental monitors for DRGs that are not only top-ranked for the hospital but that have a "significant" percentage of charges/costs attributed to the department. Such monitors may be implemented to investigate the types of services that are most frequently ordered for patients in the DRG.

d. Identify potentially inappropriate or costly ordering practices by physicians or nurses for further review and investigation by a clinical staff committee.

Example

  - After the finance department provided a list of the hospital's top 20 DRGs based on total volume of Medicare patients treated, the nurse management group in one institution requested statistical information on the utilization of nursing services for Medicare and non-Medicare patients in the top five DRGs. The nurse managers requested the:

    - Total hours of nursing care provided to patients in each of the top five DRGs

    - Total estimated nursing costs for each of the five DRGs

    This information (see Table 1) revealed that a large number of cases were classified in DRG 468 (Unrelated OR Procedure), and, as a result, these cases were reviewed by a peer review organization (PRO). The nurse management group instituted a FOCUSED MONITOR of cases assigned DRG 468 to determine if the nursing assessments, care plans and documentation were meeting PRO standards. To be sure lapses in nursing practice were not responsible for denial of payment by the PRO, the group also requested that the nurse liaison to the institution's DRG committee and an ad hoc committee of staff nurses review all cases for which payment was denied by the PRO and ascertain the:

TABLE 1:   Analysis of Nursing Costs in Top Five DRGs (by Volume) for All Discharges Between July 1 and December 31

DRG No. and Description	Total No. of Patients	Total Charges For All Services	Avg. LOS	Total Nursing Cost*	Avg. Nursing Cost Per Case*
106 Coronary Bypass with cath.	209	$5,276,974	16.4	$844,360	$4,040.00
127 Heart Failure and Shock	186	1,066,565	7.4	151,590	815.00
122 AMI, no complications, alive	145	728,465	14.0	203,000	1,400.00
243 Back disorder, Medical	109	305,667	8.6	36,842	338.00
468 Unrelated OR Procedure	104	1,079,724	12.8	154,752	1,488.00

*Nursing costs are estimated and include direct patient care time as well as time spent in activities that are indirectly related to patient care (eg, charting, care planning, order transcription, etc).

- Reason for denial

- Completeness of admission assessments by RNs

- Completeness/timeliness of nursing documentation that reflects patients' nursing care needs and their progress toward goals set in the nursing care plan

STRATEGY 2:   Creating Profiles of the Department's Top DRGs

Nurse managers who take this approach:

a. Identify the top 10 or 20 DRGs for the nursing department.

   The top DRGs may be:

   - those with the highest estimated costs for departmental services and/or

   - those whose estimated costs for departmental services represent a significant proportion of overall patient charges and/or

   - those with the highest mean nursing care hours per patient or per admission and/or

   - those with the most frequently occurring nursing diagnoses

b. Screen a sample of records of patients to identify the current mix of dependent and independent nursing functions for each DRG. These nursing functions then can be used as criteria in a FOCUSED MONITOR to disclose orders for nursing services that vary significantly from the current mix of services for a particular DRG, including:

- repeat orders for unusual services or combinations of services for patients

- unusually high or low volumes of departmental services ordered per admission

- orders for more expensive services when less expensive services would be just as effective or even more effective (eg, orders for special decubitus care when a less expensive method of treatment yields the same results)

NOTE: Variations from the current mix of services do not necessarily mean that the use of such services was inappropriate. The clinical implications of variations must be decided by the medical or nursing staff.

Examples

- In one institution, DRG 089 (Pneumonia, Pleurisy over age 69 with complications) had an average length of stay less than the state average, but the average nursing care costs per case were significantly above the mean reported by the state for that DRG.

  Since the respiratory therapy department had recently reduced its staff, the nursing DRG task force suspected that the high nursing costs might be due to the fact that nurses were performing respiratory therapy procedures during off-shifts and on weekends. The task force formed an ad hoc committee with representatives from the task force and the respiratory therapy department to collect data on patients in DRG 089 concerning the

  - Average nursing care hours per patient per day

  - Number and type of respiratory therapy procedures ordered

  - Number and type of procedures performed by respiratory therapy personnel and nursing personnel by day of the week and shift

  An analysis of the data indicated that nurses were performing respiratory therapy procedures that had been done by respiratory therapists in the past. This practice was increasing nursing care time and average nursing costs for patients in DRG 089 and, perhaps the other DRGs in the same major diagnostic category (MDC). As a result of these findings, the assistant vice-president for nursing and the director of the respiratory therapy department were able to substantiate the need for reinstituting several respiratory therapists to provide adequate coverage.

- A FOCUSED MONITOR was instituted by the professional nurse practice committee in a nursing department to evaluate the lengths of stay and the achievement of education-related goals by patients admitted to medical units with a diagnosis of diabetes mellitus. The data from the monitor suggested that the standardized nursing care plan used for these patients was no longer relevant. The stated goals were unachievable by most patients within the average length of stay designated for patients in that DRG. In some cases, patients were kept in the hospital for extra days so teaching by the nursing staff could be completed. In other instances, patients were discharged before goals were reached creating conflict between physicians and nursing staff. The nursing plan of care resulted in costly lengths of stay and the quality of the educational services to the patients was inconsistent. Based on the results of the monitor, the professional nurse practice committee revised the goals in the standardized care plan so they were more realistic for the average length of stay and more specific for the immediate needs of the patients. The goals mandated that (1) all patients with the diagnosis of diabetes mellitus would be assessed for their educational needs prior to discharge, (2) all patients with identified needs would be encouraged to permit referral to an agency for follow-up after discharge and (3) the specific educational deficit responsible for the current admission would be the primary focus of the nursing staff's educational effort during the hospitalization.

  Subsequent monitoring of the lengths of stay and goal achievement for these patients indicated that patients were being discharged in a more timely manner, thus reducing cost, yet were consistently able to meet the education-related goals specified in their plan of care.

Nurse managers who are contemplating this approach should consider the following guidelines:

- Invite and make use of input from physicians and staff nurses from the beginning. If asked to contribute to such an investigation at the outset, physicians and nurses will more likely cooperate at the end of the study when data suggest the need for more cost-efficient ordering practices.

- Collect data on DRGs for which there is a consensus among physicians and nursing staff about the range and types of services that normally should be ordered (eg, postoperative patients without complications.)

Physicians and nurses are less likely to challenge an analysis of data for such DRGs, and an analysis of this type will set the stage for reviewing other DRGs for which there may be wide variations in orders for services.

- Do not simply "adopt" patterns of practice, national or regional norms or statistics obtained from other institutions. At least initially use patterns that represent the current ordering practices in your institution. Then, if the data or your institution indicate that all or most professionals are overusing specific services and making the hospital less competitive with others in the area, you may consider using patterns of practice and statistics from other institutions to compare against your institution's performance.

- Initially review a sample of patient records in which the admitting and discharge diagnoses are straightforward and identical. A patient admitted with a vague diagnosis (eg, abdominal pain, dizziness) or one admitted with gall bladder disease and discharged with pancreatic cancer probably will receive more variable services than a patient admitted with known appendicitis or a fractured femur.

STRATEGY 3:   Monitoring the Demand for a Specific Service and Its Effect on the Hospital's Top DRGs

Nurse managers who take this approach:

a. Identify a dependent or independent nursing function that they suspect or know

  - is misused

  - has a less costly but equally effective alternative

  - may affect the profitability of a number of the hospital's top-ranked DRGs

b. Implement a monitor to determine for each of the hospital's top-ranked DRGs the:

  - total volume of orders for the specific service

  - nursing time allocated to the specific service

  - nursing costs for the specific service

c. Institute a followup monitor for the DRG(s) with the highest total volume of orders, nursing time or costs to investigate the ordering practices of physicians and nurses

d. Report to the appropriate clinical committee the effect that misuse of the service will have on profitability for the hospital's top DRGs.

Example

- The patient classification committee in nursing services in one institution noted that staff nurses were automatically ordering multi-system assessments for every patient regardless of the patient's acuity level, medical or nursing care needs or stage of illness. This practice consumed approximately 140 hours of nursing care time per day for an average census. The committee felt that changing this practice for the ten highest-volume DRGs in the institution could significantly improve the efficiency of the nursing staff and perhaps decrease costs for these DRGs. Representatives from the committee and the nursing staff of general medical/surgical units formed an ad hoc task force to collect data on the following items for one quarter:

- Number of patients in each of the hospital's top DRGs

- Total hours of nursing care given to patients in the DRG

- Total estimated nursing costs for each DRG

- Average number of multisystem assessments ordered (by shift and day) for patients in each DRG

- Average number of multisystem assessments ordered per day for each acuity level of patients in the DRG

- Total hours of nursing time spent performing multisystem assessments

- Estimated cost of performing multisystem assessments

If the monitor suggested that nursing assessments were too extensive and were increasing the cost of nursing services, the committee would turn the results over to the professional nurse practice committee, which then would be responsible for planning and implementing guidelines for appropriately ordering multisystem assessments.

Category I.   Utilization Monitors

Subcategory B: *Clinical Appropriateness and Timeliness of Admissions, Orders and Referrals*

In addition to the cost-efficient use of departmental services, nurse managers must ensure that services are appropriate to patients' clinical needs. They can detect potential problems in the appropriateness and timeliness of admissions, physicians' or nurses' orders, or referrals from other departments through their monitoring program. Managers can handle any identified problems internally by committees within the clinical unit or the department, or they may refer problems to institutional or inter-departmental committees (such as UR, safety, nursing/pharmacy committee, etc) that will identify any inappropriate ordering practices and recommend changes in these practices.

Nurse managers may elect to monitor the:

- Appropriateness of admission to a clinical unit based on the patient's nursing and medical care needs

- Appropriateness/timeliness of nursing orders for vital signs

- Timeliness of physicians' referrals to patient education programs sponsored by nursing services (such as the diabetic teaching program, cardiac rehabilitation program, etc)

- Timeliness of completion of nurse-to-nurse consultations

Because they involve an evaluation of clinical decision-making, include topics that are directly related to patient care and may involve clinical problem-solving activities, Monitors of Clinical Appropriateness and Timeliness of Admissions and Referrals have received much attention in JCAH accreditation literature, journals and surveys. Careful attention to this subcategory of utilization monitors will help the departmental monitoring program to meet JCAH QA standards.

Monitors of Clinical Appropriateness and Timeliness of Admissions, Orders and Referrals are often time-limited, and they are usually focused. Specific monitors may be recommended by nurse managers, staff nurses, clinicians on clinical committees or the QA or UR coordinator.

When choosing Monitors of Clinical Appropriateness, managers in nursing services should look at services for which the federal government, third-party payors, health maintenance organizations (HMOs) or other groups have set reimbursement guidelines that are based on documentation of the patient's need for them. Since nurses are the only professionals who monitor patients 24 hours a day, seven days a week, they are in the best position to know and report seemingly inappropriate admissions, ordering patterns or referrals and to help the hospital determine when payment most likely will be denied.

Category I: Utilization Monitors

Subcategory C: Clinicians' Use of Assessments and Recommendations Made by Staff Nurses, Clinical Nurse Specialists or Nurse Managers

These monitors seek to evaluate what many clinicians and hospital professionals believe is the most critical aspect of utilization of nursing services: use of nurses' assessments and recommendations by physicians, other nurses and professionals in other departments. Because of the close relationship between nurses and patients, the nursing staff can make meaningful evaluations of patients' ongoing needs and responses to therapeutic regimens.

Monitors in this subcategory may be initiated because clinicians *are not* (1) appropriately using the results of nursing assessments in their patient treatment decisions, (2) following nurses' recommendations on the type, sequence and timing of tests, procedures or studies, (3) considering nurses' assessments of possible contraindications for certain therapies or (4) making necessary referrals.

Monitors in this subcategory may include:

- Use of nurses' recommendations for changing drug therapy for patients who are in pain

- Use of nurses' recommendations for referring patients to aftercare agencies (such as VNA, Reach-to-Recovery, Family and Children Services, etc)

- Response by physicians to requests from nurses on the evening and night shifts for reevaluation of a patients's condition

- Response by primary nurses to clinical nurse specialists' recommendations for changing the nursing care plan for certain patients

The data for some Monitors of Clinicians' Use of Assessments and Recommendations may be retrieved from computer-based patient information systems that store test results and physicians' orders. In most hospitals, however, tracking the clinical use of assessments or recommendations will require a manual review of patient records or a log of experiences. The monitors in this subcategory are generally FOCUSED and time-limited. The data these monitors generate are usually given to a nursing committee, interdisciplinary committee or medical staff leader who have the authority to resolve problems involving clinical practice.

Because monitors in this subcategory evaluate clinical decision-making, deal with issues that directly affect patient care and may result in clinical problem-solving, they help meet JCAH QA standards.

CATEGORY II.   DEPARTMENTAL PERFORMANCE MONITORS

Measure the quality and efficiency of performance of the entire nursing department or of specific sections and functions within the department.

Data generated from Performance Monitors are used by managers and administrators in the nursing department to:

- Determine the level of efficiency of nursing operations; detect and provide objective evidence of impediments to efficient operation of the department; and track progress in improving the efficiency of departmental operations over time

- Estimate costs associated with overall operations of the nursing department as well as with specific procedures and functions performed by the department; estimate profitability of departmental operations; more accurately forecast budget requirements for the nursing department; identify aspects of departmental operations that are unnecessarily costly; decide where cost reductions can be made

- Determine staff compliance with standards of practice, regulations and policies and procedures; detect and provide evidence of impediments to staff compliance with standards of practice, regulations and policies and procedures; track progress in improving staff compliance with standards, regulations and policies and procedures

- Determine current educational needs of the nursing staff

- Provide an objective basis for staff performance appraisals, assignments, promotions, disciplinary actions, etc

- Identify potential exposure to liability by hospital or nursing staff

Category II.   Departmental Performance Monitors

Subcategory A: Overall Departmental Performance Monitors

These monitors provide a gross statistical look across a department's functions, sections and staff and are therefore SCANNING MONITORS. The statistics generated by these monitors document the quality, timeliness, volume or efficiency of nursing services across-the-board. Overall Performance Monitors are usually conducted on a continuous basis, and summary reports are compiled quarterly or semiannually. These monitors should not be continued *ad infinitum* without reappraisal, however. As with other monitors, managers should periodically assess the usefulness and reliability of the information Overall Performance Monitors provide and alter or discontinue a monitor as needed.

The summary data obtained through Overall Performance Monitors may be compared with preset goals or levels chosen by nurse managers and administrators on the basis of inhouse data or the professional literature. Some hospitals have access to performance statistics from other hospitals against which they may compare their own data.

Computer-based information systems greatly increase the efficiency with which data can be collected for these monitors. Whether or not a nurse manager makes use of a computer-based information system, he or she may wish to conduct Overall Performance Monitors of the following:

- Number of RN assessments completed within a specified time of admission of patients to general care units

- Timeliness of assignment of patients to a primary care nurse

- Estimated cost of nursing time spent in non-nursing activities

- Total and average number of nursing care hours provided by float personnel each shift

- Compliance to procedures during codes for CPR

- Reduction in rate of complications related to bedrest following inservice education program on decubitus care

- Number of nurses attending continuing education programs (by type of program)

- Number of records with incomplete documentation of nursing care (by type of personnel)

- Infection rate per unit/department (by type of infection)

- Number of malpractice cases in nursing

- Error rate in medication administration

NOTE: Some writers and consultants have suggested that a series of Overall Performance Monitors is all that a department needs for a successful monitoring program. *This simply is not the case.* In and of themselves, these monitors will not satisfy JCAH departmental monitoring requirements. More importantly, these monitors will not meet the total management information needs of a department.

Productivity

One of the key areas about which hospital managers are gathering overall performance data involves staff productivity. Productivity is a crucial measure of ongoing departmental performance, and it is especially useful for planning reductions or increases in the number or types of services offered, scheduling staff and computing departmental budgets. Productivity is such a telling indicator of performance that some hospitals are employing outside consultants or hiring inhouse management engineers to standardize the process by which productivity is defined, monitored and measured and to help department managers conduct monitors of productivity.

Despite its value, productivity has not been routinely measured in nursing. Productivity measurement is extremely difficult in nursing for a variety of reasons, including the:

- Vagueness of nursing inputs beyond the traditional "nursing care hours"

- Lack of concern about finding the least costly combination of inputs

- Vagueness of nursing outputs beyond the traditional "patient day" or hours of patient care

- Status of nursing services as intermediate rather than final services

- difficulty in measuring the effectiveness as well as the efficiency of nursing services

Because of these problems, the measurement of nursing productivity at best can yield rough estimates of departmental performance. In this book measurements of productivity are strictly quantitative. Productivity measurements may include, for example:

- Average hours of nursing care per patient day for each nursing acuity level in a patient classification system

- Average hours of nursing care per patient day for patients in a particular DRG

- Average hours of nursing care for the average length of stay for patients in a particular DRG

- Average nursing cost per patient day (or for the average length of stay) for patients in a particular DRG

- Number of nurse-sponsored education programs (eg, diabetic classes, cardiac rehabilitation classes) held per month/quarter

- Average number of parenteral infusions that are monitored by nursing staff in the department and in each clinical unit per shift/day

- Average number of admission assessments completed by each RN in the department and in each clinical unit

Establishing a Productivity Index

Most calculations of productivity for a clinical unit or the entire nursing department are rudimentary. Often productivity is calculated by dividing the nursing workload by the total number of nursing care hours available (ie, the total number of available staff) and by estimating the number of hours that were productive. The estimate of productive hours usually is determined by the nursing administration and as a rule is set at six to eight hours per direct care giver per shift.

A more standardized method of determining productivity involves a Productivity Index.

To create a Productivity Index, nurse managers should:

a. Plan and implement a reliable and valid patient classification system which converts patient care needs into hours of nursing care time required or nursing workload.

   (In absence of the complete computations needed to obtain a Productivity Index, this workload measurement can be used to estimate the personnel requirements for a department.)

b. Monitor all paid hours for direct care givers in the department or a specific clinical unit, differentiating between the hours that are directly involved in producing outputs and benefit hours (vacation, sick time, holiday, lunch hours, breaks). *

c. Approximate the total number of productive paid hours as follows:

   Productive hours = Total hours paid - Benefit hours

d. Calculate a Productivity Index as follows:

   Productivity Index = Workload/productive hours worked x 100%

* When measuring productivity, nurse managers must decide whether their units of production (ie, hours of service) will be measured in *required* hours (which are based on projected patient care requirements obtained from a patient classification system) or *provided* hours (which are based on the actual hours of nursing care delivered to a patient). These measures must be further refined to yield information on the productivity of different levels of nursing personnel.

An ideal departmental Productivity Index, of course, would be 100 percent, meaning that all staff time has been productive. Productivity Indices at times may be greater than 100 percent. These indices are artificial in the sense that individuals cannot, on an ongoing basis, produce more than "100 percent." These indices do suggest, however, that some required patient care needs have not been met during a particular shift/day.

Nurse administrators must accept the responsibility for determining satisfactory ranges of productivity and intervening when the index for a clinical unit or department is consistently over 100 percent. Although hiring additional staff is a common remedy for Productivity Indices over 100 percent, pressures for cost containment require nurse managers to explore and develop creative and effective alternatives. Nurse managers may, for example, adjust the expectations of nursing care plans and the level of required nursing care to conform to reduced lengths of stay and the shift of services from the inpatient to the outpatient sector. As nurse managers explore such alternatives, they must be careful to consult with staff nurses and physicians so the quality of care rendered by the department will not be compromised.

Although a Productivity Index allows managers to estimate productivity more reliably than before, it is limited. The Productivity Index, like data generated from other Performance Monitors, can provide only a crude or gross estimate of departmental functioning. Moreover, monitors in this subgroup cannot be used in isolation. Because they are SCANNING MONITORS, they may be used to suggest problems in the quality and efficiency of services, but they must be followed by a thorough investigative study or a FOCUSED MONITOR.

Furthermore, Productivity Indices are difficult to compare over time. Productivity Indices may vary because of fluctuations in the demand for nursing services; because of differences in the knowledge and skill level of nursing personnel, the nature of the tasks performed, the physical layout of clinical units, the materials management procedures and the equipment used; or because of disruptions in the work schedule to handle emergencies, perform some non-nursing functions or respond to other interruptions.

Category II: Departmental Performance Monitors

Subcategory B   Performance of Specific Departmental Functions Involving Direct Patient Care

This subcategory of Performance Monitors is the most familiar to nurse managers. Nurse managers put in place monitors of this type to satisfy department-specific QA standards of the JCAH and to assess the accuracy, timeliness or efficiency with which nursing services are carried out on each clinical unit, during each shift or for each nursing function on a clinical unit.

Monitors of Specific Departmental Functions Involving Direct-Patient Care produce data similar to those generated by Overall Performance Monitors. Rather than collecting and evaluating data for the entire department, however, these monitors look at specific units, functions or procedures. Monitors of Specific Departmental Functions—Direct Patient Care involve the same calculations of productivity as the Overall Performance Monitors. Using the methodology described for the previous subgroup of monitors, a nurse manager would compute a Productivity Index for each function or unit within the department. Monitoring topics on the distribution of departmental resources in Subcategory C of this category are also related to the quantitative measurement of productivity.

Monitors of Specific Departmental Functions—Direct Patient Care may be continuous SCANNING MONITORS or FOCUSED MONITORS that are implemented on a time-limited basis to investigate a problem suggested by a SCANNING MONITOR: for example:

SCANNING MONITOR	FOCUSED MONITOR
Adherence of nursing personnel to written standards of care (by unit/ department personnel category)	Adherence of nursing personnel to written standards of care for treating patients who are considered to be at high risk for falls
Completeness of assessment of pain for postoperative patients	Completeness of assessment of pain for patients in the recovery room
Appropriateness of nursing assessment and intervention to maintain/ establish regular elimination patterns in patients	Initiation of appropriate nursing intervention to prevent/treat fecal impactions in patients having barium enema x-rays

FOCUSED MONITORS in this subcategory assess specific nursing care given to patients. As a result, they meet the basic JCAH requirement for QA monitoring. These monitors meet another JCAH QA monitoring requirement. JCAH guidelines for QA monitoring and for an integrated QA program in hospitals mandate the effective coordination of services among departments and professionals caring for patients. Monitors of Departmental Performance—Direct Patient Care can help determine to what extent patient care is being effectively coordinated. Monitors of the coordination of patient care among disciplines do, of course, require that nursing services work with targeted departments or professionals to:

- Identify the specific topics

- Set the specifications of the monitor

- Assist in data collection and analysis

- Plan and implement changes in performance if needed

FOCUSED MONITORS in this subcategory also can be used to assess the proficiency of nursing staff members. Periodic appraisal of staff competence has been a requisite for all departmental managers for years. Until recently, however, these appraisals were not done consistently, nor were they based on objective criteria. Greater accountability for objective appraisal of staff and peer review programs have prompted nurse managers to plan and implement monitors with which to evaluate staff performance. Such monitors may involve on-site observation by peers or supervisors, self-reporting by staff or a periodic review of documentation.

Organizing Monitors of Direct Patient Care

Because there are a great many potential monitors in the area of direct patient care, nurse managers must organize these monitors so they provide a comprehensive data base for use by the nursing staff and by accrediting and regulatory agencies. One method of organizing Monitors of Direct Patient Care is to categorize the monitors according to the steps of the nursing process. Thus, there will be Monitors of Direct Patient Care that are related to assessment (including nursing diagnosis), planning, implementation and evaluation (patient outcomes).

Monitors related to assessment include the accuracy, completeness, appropriateness and timeliness with which nurses collect data on patients.

Examples:

- Adequacy/completeness of assessment of the patient's condition on admission to the unit

- Accuracy of nurses' identification of deviations from established physical/emotional norms for specific types of patients

- Accuracy of nursing diagnoses for patients in DRG 127 (Heart Failure and Shock) based on the nursing assessment and nursing progress notes

- Collaboration between nursing and dietary personnel in the nutritional assessment of oncology patients

Monitors related to planning address the accuracy, completeness, appropriateness and timeliness of the written care plan which is created for a patient by nursing personnel.

Examples

- Appropriateness of goals and actions given the patient's condition and expected length of stay

- Congruence of the nursing care plan with the goals of treatment and expectations of the patient

- Appropriateness of nursing orders for intervention during certain drug regimens (eg, blood pressure monitoring of patients who are receiving antihypertensives, weight gain or loss and intake and output evaluation for patients who are receiving diuretics, etc)

- Coordination by physicians and nurses in conducting discharge planning for the patient

Monitors related to implementation focus on the adherence of nursing staff to the plan of care, to the policies and procedures for therapeutic measures they perform in implementing the plan of care and the skill they demonstrate during the performance of the procedures.

Examples

- Adequacy of hygiene measures performed for patients (eg, mouth care, hair and nail care, skin care, etc)

- Adherence to written standards of care for the admission, transfer or discharge of a patient

- Maintenance of aseptic technique during procedures requiring sterility (eg, preparation of parenteral medications, dressing changes, catheterizations, etc)

- Continuation of activities by nursing personnel that support attainment of patients' physical therapy goals

Monitors related to evaluation include those which address the effects of nursing care on patient outcomes

Examples

- Patient achievement/non-achievement of predetermined goals

- Effectiveness of nursing interventions to relieve pain in post-surgical patients

- Rate of readmission of diabetic patients within 60 days of discharge for treatment of a condition related to diabetic therapy

- Adequacy of preparation of patients for GI series

Monitors related to evaluation can also be used to evaluate retrospectively the efficacy of nursing judgments that can affect patient outcomes. Such monitors most closely address the professional management of patient care by nursing staff. These monitors focus on issues that can arise despite the adherence of nursing staff to policies and procedures of assessment, planning and implementation of the plan of care.

Example

- In one institution, an elderly patient developed a severe impaction following a barium enema and had to undergo surgery for its removal. The hospital QA committee, in reviewing the case, determined that the nursing staff had assessed the patient's ongoing constipation, had planned appropriate measures to relieve it, and had implemented these measures as well as the physician's orders for laxatives and enemas. The conclusion of the committee was that the patient's hypoactive bowel was the reason for the impaction and that the medical and nursing staffs had done all they could to rectify the situation.

  A monitor evaluating the judgments of the nursing staff would have had a different approach. The monitor would have focused on why the initial nursing assessment of the elimination pattern in this patient did not prompt the nurse to suggest that the physician reconsider the use of the barium enema as a diagnostic test in this high-risk patient. Both the nursing judgment of what to assess for this patient and how to best use the data gathered in the assessment to prevent an untoward patient outcome would have been part of the monitoring process.

Other examples

- Appropriateness/timeliness of nursing interventions for patients suffering nausea and vomiting as a side effect from radiation or drug therapy

- Timeliness of nursing interventions for patients susceptible to/experiencing nutritional deficiencies

- Appropriateness of written discharge information to patients

Category II.   Departmental Performance Monitors

Subcategory C: Availability, Distribution and Appropriateness of Use of Departmental Resources

This subcategory of Departmental Performance Monitors is implemented to determine whether staffing, equipment and supply levels meet demands for service in each clinical unit, for each function and during each shift. Monitors in this subcategory also may be implemented to track staffing issues such as absenteeism and turnover.

Many departments have instituted Monitors of Use of Resources to evaluate the appropriateness of staff use of supplies and equipment. Under prospective pricing and internal and external cost-containment programs, managers must demonstrate that they are economical and judicious in their assessments of staff and in the use of resources. Furthermore, they must objectively demonstrate increased demands for services or threats to the quality of service before adding staff or new equipment. As with other Performance Monitors, monitors in this subcategory may include continuous SCANNING MONITORS as well as time-limited FOCUSED MONITORS of such topics as:

- Ratio of FTEs: Surgery cases in all surgery suites by time of day, by day and by week

- Availability of float personnel to meet nursing staff shortages on off hours and weekends

- Appropriateness of assignment of nursing personnel based on nursing care needs of the patient, acuity data and institutional policies

- Utilization of LPNs for specialized procedures on specific units or in the department

- Turnover rate for stock medications/supplies on the unit

- Adequacy of clean linen supply in patient care units

- Availability of equipment needed for specific unit procedures (eg, cutdown trays, tracheostomy trays, thoracotomy trays, etc)

Category II.   Departmental Performance Monitors

Subcategory D.   Documentation

The necessity for clear, concise, accurate and complete documentation of patient care by nursing personnel has been addressed in the literature, in continuing education programs, in nursing QA programs and risk management efforts. Added to the variety of reasons used to demonstrate the need for pertinent documentation in the past are new pressures for timely and precise documentation to comply with the prospective pricing system and PROs.

Under the prospective pricing system, the adequacy of documentation determines the amount that hospitals will receive for treating patients. Lack of documentation of the patient's needs and the services that were rendered may cause the fiscal, intermediary to place the patient in a lower-paying DRG or the PRO to deny reimbursement for certain days of stay or for a readmission if the PRO believes hospitalization was unnecessary.

Moreover, inaccurate information on charges for equipment and supplies used by patients may distort the actual costs of treating patients in a DRG.

The adequacy of documentation also can foster the expeditious discharge of patients, which is crucial under prospective pricing to assure that the cost of the patient's stay does not exceed set reimbursement levels and, if possible, to reduce the cost of the patient's hospitalization. Delayed or inaccurate documentation can interfere with evaluations of the efficacy of the patient's treatment plan, identification of potential complications and the institution of discharge planning.

Monitors of Documentation may be undertaken to (1) assure that documentation by the nursing staff is complete, timely and accurate, (2) help other professionals identify gaps in documentation that affect the reimbursement the hospital will obtain or lengthen the patient's hospitalization, (3) check on the appropriateness of charge information and (4) assess compliance to the procedures for determining charges.

These monitors can be used to evaluate the information about aftercare that nurses give to patients or agencies to whom patients are referred. With the heightened involvement of the consumer in his/her health care and the increased use of outpatient health care delivery systems, nursing staff in hospitals are providing greater amounts of written information that will be used by patients long after discharge. Because this phenomenon has implications involving both quality assurance and risk management, nurse managers will want to monitor aftercare instructions to be sure they are given at the proper time and that they are clear and accurate.

Monitors in the subcategory of Documentation may be SCANNING or FOCUSED, and they may cover such topics as:

- Accuracy of documentation of admission of a woman in labor, including notation of:

    -any rupture of the membranes
    -uterine tone and contractions

-evaluation of blood loss
-gestational age
-previous pregnancies and outcomes

- Documentation of reasons why ordered medications were not given

- Accuracy/completeness of documentation of IV therapy

- Accuracy/completeness of documentation of medically prescribed treatments for patients

- Documentation of diabetic patients' knowledge of self-care prior to discharge

- Accuracy/completeness of written discharge information given to patients

- Accuracy of charges for IV fluids

CATEGORY III.   USER SATISFACTION MONITORS

Measure the perceptions of the adequacy of departmental services held by physicians, patients, patient family members and hospital staff

---

As hospital administrators and managers developed QA/RM programs over the last ten years, they came to realize the importance of input from the individuals they serve. Administrators and managers have found that surveys, questionnaires, interviews and reviews of complaints uncover problems and concerns that would not come to light through traditional evaluation techniques.

User Satisfacton Monitors obtain individuals' perceptions of efficiency, quality and timeliness of services, the environment in which the services are delivered and the personal characteristics of the staff (warmth, concern, helpfulness).

Information generated from User Satisfaction Monitors can be used by administrators and nurse managers to identify:

- User dissatisfaction with the quality, timeliness, or nature of services provided

- Actual improvements in the quality, timeliness or nature of services

- Ways to inform physicians and/or patients of new services

- Potential sources of legal claims against the institution or nursing staff

- Ways to enhance the image of the hospital in the community

There is wide variance in the frequency of User Satisfaction Monitors. Most hospitals administer periodically throughout the year general surveys and questionnaires for several departments and services to scan a wide range of topics related to user satisfaction. Complaints and suggestions are collected continuously and summarized on a quarterly or semiannual basis. The results of these SCANNING MONITORS may suggest the need for more FOCUSED MONITORS of specific problem areas. As with other User Satisfaction Monitors, user satisfaction surveys should not be continued *ad infinitum;* they should be reappraised at least every six months. They may cover such topics as:

- Patient satisfaction with the timeliness of treatment by the triage nurse in the emergency department

- Family members' (or significant others') satisfaction with the degree to which they were informed of the progress of the patient during surgery and the recovery period

- Physician satisfaction with the diabetic education program for their patients

- Patient satisfaction with the response of nursing personnel to requests for pain relievers

---

CATEGORY IV.   SAFETY MONITORS

Review the environment in which departmental procedures are performed, the potential and known hazards to patients and staff and the readiness of staff to recognize and respond to hazards.

Information generated from Safety Monitors is used to:

- Meet the standards of accreditation bodies, professional organizations and regulatory agencies

- Detect, evaluate and track hazards to patients and staff

Safety Monitors detect immediate dangers to the health and well-being of staff and patients resulting from exposure to flammable, radioactive, explosive or toxic substances used in the department. They also disclose other hazards, such as slippery floors and loose railings and evaluate staff preparedness for emergencies (fire or disaster). Safety Monitors may be SCANNING, FOCUSED or both. Monitors in this subgroup usually are conducted through on-site observation and testing by department staff or hospital safety personnel. Data generally are collected at specified or random periods throughout the year. The frequency of evaluation of staff preparedness is specified by standards and regulations, and observations of departmental performance must be compared with preestablished criteria.

These monitors may include:

- Adherence of nursing staff to precautions when dealing with patients who are receiving oxygen

- Appropriateness and timeliness of staff performance during fire drills

- Nursing personnel's exposure to cytotoxic agents

- Appropriateness and timeliness of staff performance during disaster drills

- Appropriate use of siderails for specific patient populations (eg, semi-conscious, elderly, sedated, etc)

CATEGORY V: QUALITY CONTROL MONITORS

Review the attainment and maintenance of expected credentialing and skill levels by departmental personnel. They also review the quality of equipment and supplies used in the course of providing services.

Information generated from Quality Control Monitors is used to:

- Meet the standards of accrediting bodies, professional organizations and regulatory agencies

- Detect and evaluate problems that may affect the reliability and accuracy of nursing services

- Track progress in resolving problems affecting the reliability and accuracy of services

Quality Control Monitors frequently are FOCUSED because they review compliance to routine expectations for personnel performance, well-established protocols and specific functional aspects of equipment and supplies. Many of these monitors have been defined in the published standards of professional organizations and accrediting and regulatory agencies. Quality Control Monitors may involve regular surveys, checklists or inspections. Often, department managers do not "take credit" for Quality Control Monitors because these monitors do not seem to be directly related to quality assurance per se, have not been recognized by the JCAH and are not consistently documented and reviewed to detect patterns of performance or problem areas. These monitors, nonetheless, are integral to the maintenance of high levels of staff performance in the care of patients.

Quality Control Monitors may be conducted on a fixed schedule during each shift, each day or each week, and they may be considered part of the customary responsibilities of nursing staff. They may cover such topics as:

- Review/revision of the policies and procedures for direct patient care for the unit or the entire department

- Timeliness of required performance appraisals for unit staff nurses

- Maintenance of updated skills inventory on all nursing staff on a clinical unit

- Verification of current licensure of all RNs and LPNs

- Verification of ACLS completion by all RNs in the emergency room within six months of assignment to the department

- Condition of brakes on beds, stretchers and wheelchairs in a unit

- Timeliness of reporting of faulty or inoperative equipment

- Availability of appropriate and functional emergency respiratory and cardiac equipment in a unit

- Thoroughness of crash cart checks per shift/day

- Maintenance of weekly microbial counts for OR suites

CATEGORY VI.   INCIDENT/OCCURRENCE MONITORS

Review episodes of actual or potential patient or employee harm.

Information generated by Incident/Occurrence Monitors may be used by department managers and administrators to:

- Identify potential claims against the facility and its staff that may arise from negligence of department staff

- Detect immediate problems in facility management and clinical practice that may endanger patient welfare

Incident/Occurrence Monitors are by no means the only risk management data-gathering activities that should be conducted at the departmental level. In fact, information collected for other monitors should be transferred to a department's liability prevention/ risk management effort. It is well established that inappropriate clinical practices, deficient performance by nursing staff, inadequate quality control of equipment and supplies and dissatisfied patients all pose a potential for liability. Therefore, Monitors of Departmental Performance, User Satisfaction, Safety and Quality Control are believed by many hospital managers to be the cornerstones of liability prevention. This fact is often overlooked by risk management consultants, who tend to promote Incident/ Occurrence Monitoring (sometimes ambiguously referred to as generic screening) to the exclusion of other valuable techniques. Incident/Occurrence Monitors are, nonetheless, critical additions to the departmental monitoring effort because they isolate actual or potential episodes of patient harm or staff negligence that may never surface otherwise.

For a number of years, Incident/Occurrence Monitors were limited to episodes that reflected problems in physician practice. In recent years, these monitors have been extended to the practice of other professionals, especially nursing, and to entire departments. In this type of monitoring activity, medical records and other documentation are screened on an ongoing basis to detect predefined "occurrences." Any identified occurrences are then summarized according to their patterns on a monthly or quarterly basis.

Predefined occurrences should be selected by the hospital risk manager and the nurse manager. Predefined occurrences can be based on lists of commonly used Incident/

Occurrence Monitors in hospital literature. They should be modified, however, to select monitors that are most relevant to nursing. Incident/Occurrence Monitors may include both SCANNING and FOCUSED MONITORS. SCANNING MONITORS (eg, the overall rate of medication errors) may reveal a problem that should be reviewed indepth using a FOCUSED MONITOR (eg, the types/causes of medication errors). Examples of these monitors may include:

- Readmission of patients within 60 days of discharge to treat complications related to the previous hospitalization

- Rate of falls in a unit/or the entire department by:

  -patient age
  -DRG classification or
  -patient acuity level

- Rate of nosocomial infections by department, unit, physician and DRG

- Performance of procedures *outside* the scope of practice of nursing personnel (eg, a nursing assistant monitoring IV therapy

- Rate of employee injuries (by type of injury for each unit and for the entire department)

- Rate of complications among patients who receive blood products

---

CATEGORY VII: MONITORS OF PATIENT MANAGEMENT AND CLINICAL PRACTICES OF OTHER DEPARTMENTS

Measure the performance of the staff of other departments or the quality and accuracy of the services which the department provides and which affect the performance and operations of the nursing department.

Because of the close interaction of nursing services with other departments and physicians, this category is uniquely relevant to the nursing department and is usually not found in the categories of monitors for other clinical departments. Usually the monitors in this category are FOCUSED MONITORS because they address specific functions of a department or the performance of its staff. These monitors help meet JCAH guidelines by promoting an integrated approach to monitoring topics related to patient care that are shared by departments in the institution.

In implementing these monitors, nursing collaborates in the evaluation of the performance of other disciplines. Nursing is, in fact, in the best position to collect data on patient care performed by others. Often, monitors in this category are conducted by interdepartmental committees or task forces that receive the data from the nursing department and then summarize, evaluate and act on the information as necessary. Some examples of these monitors are:

- Use of cephalosporins in patients who have no culture and sensitivity (C&S) report or whose C & S indicates that a low cost drug would be effective

- Accuracy of diets delivered to patients by the dietary department

When the performance of others influences performance and operation of nursing services, nurse managers can use the information generated by Monitors of Patient Management to negotiate needed changes. Examples of these types of monitors include:

- Timeliness of transferring patients to and from clinical units and other departments for surgery, tests, procedures or therapy

- Timeliness of availability of unit dose medications for administration to patients

- Turnaround time for reports of STAT laboratory tests

- Availability of equipment for continued patient therapy in departments other than nursing (i.e. suction equipment, IV poles, oxygen, etc)

Summary

Chapter 4 completes the introduction to the basic information about the concept and structure of a monitor which nurse managers need to understand in order to create a comprehensive monitoring program. Chapter 5 serves as a transition for nurse managers as they move from this general knowledge of monitors to selecting specific topics for monitors and building an Agenda of Department Monitors. Chapter 5 discusses how to integrate a monitoring program into the daily operations of the nursing department.

5: Integrating the Monitoring Activity into the "80-Hour Week"

Planning and implementing a comprehensive monitoring system when existing resources have been stretched beyond reasonable limits is a major concern for nurse managers. In a standard work week, nurse managers must respond to the demands placed upon them by hospital administration, the nursing profession, physicians, consumers and the employees for whom they are directly responsible. To integrate monitoring into this work week, which already seems to be 80 hours long, may appear to be an insurmountable task, even for the most committed professionals. However, nurse managers must successfully accomplish this task to maintain the quality of nursing care and the integrity of the nursing department in this time of cost containment.

Freeing Up Resources

Every day, nurse managers and staff decide how they will allocate their time and energy to fulfill organizational and personal goals. The institution of a comprehensive monitoring system presupposes that all members of the department will be willing to evaluate and adjust their current priorities so resources needed for the monitoring effort will become available. This reordering of priorities in the nursing department is difficult but necessary to assure that the monitoring program will continue long after its first six months or the "honeymoon phase."

The monitoring effort cannot simply be another "add-on" to existing schedules that are already too heavy. Instead, it must replace habitual, routine and comfortable activities that are inappropriate or unnecessary for functioning in the changing environment of today's hospital.

Evaluating Present Responsibilities

Before beginning the monitoring effort, nurse managers therefore must critically evaluate their current responsibilities and those of their staff and decide:

- Which activities can be "let go"

- Which activities can be shifted to other personnel within the nursing department or to other departments within the hospital

- What changes can be made in the current utilization of personnel to enhance available productive time

For example, nurse managers of clinical units often "fill in" as staff nurses when there is insufficient coverage to adequately meet patients' demand. Although a critical shortage of nursing staff can happen from time to time, in some institutions this practice is the *modus operandi* for certain clinical units, and managers' legitimate responsibilities are regularly left unattended. Increasing staffing levels and improving scheduling will resolve such misuse of resources and allow nurse managers to direct their energies toward their management functions, which include monitoring.

Staff nurses often deliver and pick up meal trays, act as messengers to carry dispatches to and from other departments or serve as furniture-and-transport personnel for multiple patient transfers. Shifting the responsibilitiy for these activities from the professional nursing staff to nonprofessional staff in another, more appropriate department will improve cost-effectiveness and free-up time for monitoring.

Analysis of the work flow during various shifts may reveal non-productive time which can be used for monitoring activities. In one institution, for example, night shift personnel were observed knitting or playing cards when things were "quiet," and nurses who worked 10-hour shifts frequently spent their overlap time doing routine charting rather than the activities that are usually neglected during the traditional 8-hour shift. Nurse managers of these units decided to redirect the energies of the staff, and with input from staff nurses, they instituted guidelines for performing nursing tasks that included monitoring activies during night shifts and 10-hour shifts. Reorganizing nurses' time yielded rewards for the organization, the employees and, most importantly, the patients.

Involving All Professional Staff in Monitoring

The success of the monitoring effort in nursing depends on the participation of *all* professional staff. Nonetheless, because nurse managers are ultimately responsible for the quality of nursing care delivered in their assigned area, they believe they must *personally* conduct the monitoring activities. If nurse managers try to do monitoring on their own, they may actually subvert the activity. Monitoring can be nebulous, even threatening, if it is imposed by some appointed group or person without the involvement of the staff on the operational "side" of the organization. Nursing staff will not understand their place in quality assurance unless they are integrally involved in the monitoring process. The quality of care that patients receive is in the hands of the nursing staff, not the managers. The staff can more fully understand this reality if they are involved in the monitoring effort of the nursing department from the outset.

Staff nurses' participation in the monitoring program also increases the resources nurse managers can tap. Professional staff nurses can become involved in the monitoring effort in a variety of ways. They can:

- Generate ideas for monitoring topics

    Staff nurses and nurse managers may have different concerns about the factors that affect the utilization and quality of nursing care. If nurse managers are the sole source of monitoring topics, important issues may be overlooked.

- Select high-priority topics

- Develop specifications for monitors

- Collect and summarize data

- Report the results of a monitor to various committees

- Participate in the resolution of problems identified by the monitoring process

Educating Staff About Monitoring

Before nurse managers can engage the professional staff in monitoring, they must be sure staff understand exactly what monitoring means. The concept of monitoring should be presented in a formal educational program that stresses the relevance of monitoring in the day-to-day performance of the department. The program should show nurses that monitoring can assist them to:

- Make the *correct* decision regarding the nursing care that should be delivered to patients on their unit

- Assure that the actions taken to implement these decisions are done correctly

The program also should point out that monitoring is a feedback mechanism for nurses and managers on their performance. It demonstrates what they do well and where they can improve.

Monitoring tasks will not attract high-priority status and substantial effort from nurse managers and staff unless the benefits of monitoring have been clearly delineated. The educational program therefore should emphasize that monitoring is essential to the nursing department for these reasons:

1. It enhances the quality of the department's services, which are an integral part of the "product" of the hospital.

2. It demonstrates professional nurses' commitment to deliver timely, appropriate and cost-effective care to consumers.

3. It stimulates the achievement of high levels of performance by nurse managers and staff.

4. It promotes participative management by encouraging the active involvement of staff nurses in the evaluation of the quality of their services and the resolution of problems that affect quality.

5. It meets the requirements of JCAH and other regulatory and accrediting agencies.

Any effort to educate individuals should build on previous knowledge, use familiar terms and relate the new knowledge to important parts of the individuals' customary work life. The steps of the nursing process can be used as an educational framework to present monitoring from a meaningful perspective. (See Chapter 6 for an explanation of how the nursing process helps organize monitoring topics.) The nursing diagnosis, which many nurses feel is vital to the establishment of a sound base for professional practice, or professional standards of practice also can be used to place monitoring topics in context.

Decentralization of the Monitoring Program

An effective way to involve professional staff in the monitoring program is to decentralize the monitoring process. By decentralizing the monitoring program to the "grass roots" or unit level, nurse managers assure that patient care problems will be recognized and resolved by those who are responsible for the delivery of the patient care. The decentralization of the monitoring effort also heightens the nursing staff's awareness of problems in the department and may prompt quick resolution of suspected or known problems.

Responsibility at the unit level may be assigned to a new monitoring team or committee, a quality circle or an existing unit committee. Monitoring should be done by individual clinical units or a cluster of units that share common interests (eg, all critical care units, all units whose patient populations primarily include children, all units that treat elderly adults who have chronic as well as acute illnesses). These clusters may also follow traditional medical models, such as:

- All medical units

- All surgical units

- Maternal/child health units

- Operating room/recovery room units

- Psychiatric/mental health units

- Short stay units

- Rehabilitation units

Despite the advantages of a decentralized monitoring program, some aspects of monitoring must be centralized to improve efficiency and effectiveness. Centralized functions:

- Prevent duplication of effort (particularly in the collection of data)

- Assure that overall departmental priorities are being addressed

- Keep the "big picture" in mind (eg, a topic of little concern in many different units may build to a "big" concern for the department)

- Coordinate department-wide monitors

- Provide an identifiable means for coordinating the nursing monitoring effort with the monitoring programs of other departments and the hospital

The Importance of the QA Coordinator and Committee

The individuals who perform centralized monitoring functions in most nursing departents are the QA coordinator in nursing and the nursing QA committee. Because of cost-containment pressures, administrators in some institutions have eliminated the position of QA coordinator and/or distributed QA duties among several nurse managers. Fragmentation of the QA effort in nursing may be workable in a small hospital; however, in most institutions, it will result in a disorganized, duplicative and ineffective monitoring program in nursing services.

Hospital administrators and nurse managers may have difficulty understanding and justifying the need for a QA coordinator in nursing in a decentralized monitoring system. However, they need only look at other industries that have cut back on quality assurance efforts to readily identify the long-term ramifications of such decisions. The retention of a central QA coordinator in nursing as well as a central QA committee is highly recommended because of the many critical responsibiiities they would assume including:

- Teaching QA skills to nurse managers and staff

- Orienting new managers and staff to the monitoring program and the roles they will play in it

- Evaluating the monitoring program

- Resolving problems in the implementation of the program

- Facilitating interdepartmental monitors

- Meshing the nursing QA program with the hospital-wide program

The effectiveness and efficiency of the monitoring program in the nursing department can be enhanced in other ways as well. As pointed out in Chapter 2, nurse managers can identify and use existing data bases in the institution. Nurse managers must institute effective communication systems with other departments to learn what data are available and how their use in nursing can be facilitated.

Making Monitoring Part of the Nursing Department's Routine

Monitoring activities should be done in conjunction with other departmental duties as much as possible so monitors can become part of the day-to-day functions of the department. Collection of data for monitors can become part of the "routine" of nurse managers and staff alike. As managers make "rounds" on their respective units and receive reports from employees, they can collect data on topics that have been selected for monitors. Nursing staff can be expected to incorporate monitoring activities into their weekly work schedule, and clinical committees can make some aspect of the monitoring process a regular part of their agenda.

Examples

- The head nurse of a unit had been told by a concerned staff nurse that patients were not receiving proper mouth care. As part of the monitoring effort to validate this concern, the head nurse decided to conduct short interviews with patients on their mouth care and observe the condition of the mouths of selected patients during her rounds on the unit.

- The staff nurses on the night shift in one unit were given a specified number of medical records to review each month as part of a monitor to evaluate written nursing care plans for patients and documentation of patients' progress toward their treatment goals.

- In one institution, part of the monthly staff meeting on the clinical unit was set aside for monitoring activities, including data collection via medical record review, compilation of summary reports, analysis of completed reports and discussion of plans for resolving identified problems.

- As part of their regular duties, interdepartmental committees in one facility followed-up on monitors that were identified by clinical units and the nursing QA committee.

In addition to incorporating monitoring into the daily operations of the department, nurse managers can use the data collected through monitors to fulfill other responsibilities. For example, monitors can provide data for:

- Performance appraisals

- Strategic and long range planning

- Creation of relevant education programs

Establishing Controls

Nurse managers will want to establish controls on their monitoring system during the initial phases of planning and implementation. These controls are necessary to ensure that the program will remain a realistic, ongoing part of the department's efforts to provide high-quality care within limited resources.

These controls involve selecting only high-priority topics for monitoring, matching monitoring efforts and available institutional resources and continually evaluating the monitoring activity. Monitoring must not become a rote exercise in data collection. The information provided by monitors must prompt action, such as:

- Decision to "drop" monitors that are no longer necessary

- Movement toward indepth investigation and resolution of an identified problem

- Replacement of existing or outdated monitors with more important and timely ones

Summary

To integrate a comprehensive monitoring program into the "80-hour" nursing work week, nurse managers must:

- Evaluate present management and staff functions and reallocate staff time to address high-priority activities, including monitoring.

- Involve all levels of nursing personnel in the monitoring program to assure that pertinent topics are selected and high-priority issues are identified and addressed

- Educate managers and staff using familiar and important concepts, such as the nursing process and nursing diagnosis, to enhance understanding of monitoring and its relevance to the professional work role

- Centralize selected monitoring functions to reduce duplication of effort and coordinate intra and interdepartmental monitoring efforts

- Utilize existing data bases and personnel in various departments that can be helpful in the department's monitoring program

- Dovetail data collection and dissemination into the existing "routine" and structure of the department's day-to-day operations

- Create a realistic, dynamic monitoring program which provides feedback to professional nurses on their performance and stimulates action needed to achieve high-quality services

As nurse managers select topics for monitors, delineate the specifications for the chosen monitors and develop an Agenda of Monitors, they can apply the concepts from this chapter to assure that their monitoring program will be workable in *their* institutions.

6: Choosing Topics for Monitors

With an understanding of the structure, types and categories of monitors (as presented in Chapters 3 and 4) and the integration of the monitoring process in nursing services (as presented in Chapter 5), nurse managers can now direct their attention to the selection of monitoring topics for each clinical area and the department as a whole. This chapter presents for each category of monitors, lists of topics that are representative of ongoing monitoring efforts in nursing services. However, the lists do not include *all possible* topics or all the topics that are *currently being monitored* by nursing departments. Moreover, the lists of monitors are not intended to be adopted wholesale, but to provide "food for thought" as nurse managers plan their own individualized programs.

Many suggested topics in this chapter are narrow in focus. These topics illustrate the level of specificity with which a topic should be stated so it can be clearly understood and managed in terms of data collection. Examples of these kinds of topics include:

- Capability of oncology patients to perform self-care with Hickman catheters at time of discharge

- Nurses' assessment of specified high-risk factors to identify patients who need discharge planning

- Competence of unit personnel in obtaining accurate lying and standing blood pressure readings

Other suggested topics are broad or cover multiple monitoring areas. Nurse managers therefore will want to refine topic statements so the topics relate specifically to their institution. For example, one topic covers the average number of special therapies ordered (by type of therapy and unit) including:

- Tracheostomies

- Enteral feedings

- Total parenteral nutrition (TPN)

- Central venous pressure (CVP) monitoring

- Intraaortic balloon pump (IABP)

- Weight per bed scales

- Lidocaine/streptokinase drips

A nurse manager will want to choose only those few special therapies that (1) are currently affecting the utilization of nursing personnel in the institution or (2) may have a major impact on the department in the future.

Although many topics may initially appear to be too global, complex or concentrated for an individual monitoring effort, nurse managers must keep in mind that the selection of a "wish list" of topics for each clinical area and the overall department is *just a beginning step* in the process of developing an Agenda of Department Monitors. Subsequent decisions on the variables (data) and frequency and amount of data to be collected will determine the parameters of the topics selected. For example, nurse managers may choose topics because data can be obtained from computerized data bases or by clerical personnel. Such topics may include:

- Statistical distribution of the top 25 DRGs in the department by volume of patients

- Turnaround time between the patient's request for pain medication and the administration of the medication by nursing personnel

- Number of falls by patients over age 65 that occurred in each unit or in the entire department

When compiling a list of monitoring topics, nurse managers must:

- Evaluate their current monitoring program to determine what monitors should be added, deleted or changed

- Decide which monitors will have the biggest "payoff" for their department and the hospital

This chapter will help nurse managers accomplish the first objective. The second objective will be addressed in Chapter 7.

Evaluating the Current Monitoring Program

Every hospital department has a monitoring program to meet JCAH standards or the requirements of regulatory agencies and professional organizations. By building on this monitoring effort, each department manager can develop a comprehensive monitoring program that will meet specific departmental needs and goals.

The Unit/Department Monitoring Profile (see the form on page 74) can help managers analyze their present monitoring endeavors. This form should be used to:

- Identify, for each category and subcategory of monitor, the monitors that are currently being undertaken within the department or those being done inside and outside the department

- Decide which topics of monitors should be added to or substituted for current monitors, using the lists of suggested topics in this chapter as a base

- Specify whether or not selected topics are a priority, using the guidelines in Chapter 7

In most hospitals the Monitoring Profile cannot be completed soley by nurse managers because a considerable amount of monitoring is done outside individual clinical units or the overall nursing department. In many cases nurse managers may not even be aware of all the present or planned monitoring that concerns their department's services. Nurse managers therefore must collaborate with a number of individuals or committees, such as the nursing QA coordinator/committee, hospital QA administrator, risk manager, UR coordinator, members of the UR and other medical staff evaluation committees, financial and billing managers, data processing staff, safety engineer and the DRG/case-mix coordinator. Nurse managers also may wish to work with the hospital administration and management engineers who may be consulting with other hospital departments, and they may seek input from supervisors and staff from each clinical area and shift. Completion of the Monitoring Profile thus may involve a series of meetings and discussions, informal and formal, over a number of weeks.

Once nurse managers have assessed the scope of current monitors, they and their staff must decide what other monitors would offer critical, pertinent information about the functioning of the nursing department. To assist managers in this arduous process, a sample of monitoring topics which reflect current reimbursement, cost containment, quality assurance, user satisfaction, safety, quality control and professional liability issues follows the topics were derived from interviews and surveys of nurse managers, nursing QA specialists, hospital QA coordinators and risk managers as well as a review of the professional nursing literature. The topics are divided into the seven major categories and their subcategories that were outlined in Chapter 4. These topics by no means represent all the possible monitoring topics for these categories. They do, however, illustrate the common concerns of many nursing services today. (See Chapter 4 for a discussion of each category and the factors that go into the selection of topics for each category).

Unit/Department Monitoring Profile

CATEGORY:

Subcategory:

CURRENT TOPICS BEING MONITORED	CONTINUE?		ALTERNATIVE/ ADDITIONAL TOPICS	PRIORITY?	
	Yes	No		Yes	No

Sample Monitoring Topics

Category I.   Utilization Monitors

Subcategory A: Statistical Distribution Related to Orders, Referrals and Costs

Topics:

- Total and average number of admissions/discharges (by unit) for the entire department

- Total and average number of admissions (by hour/shift/day of the week) for each unit

- Average daily census by unit and for the entire department

- Total number of patients treated on each clinical unit by:

  -DRG
  -payor category

- Distribution of the patient population in each unit by:

  -age
  -payor category
  -sex
  -race
  -residence (zip code)

- Homogeneity of the patient mix on each clinical unit based on the following characteristics:

  -medical care requirements
  -nursing care requirements
  -procedures ordered
  -special skills needed by staff

- Number of patients in each nursing diagnosis (by clinical unit)

- Total and average number of physicians' orders for nursing services per patient (by unit)

- Number of patient contacts generated by physicians' orders by type of personnel (ie, licensed and unlicensed) in each unit

- Total and average number of nursing orders for nursing services (per patient) for the 10 DRGs that have the highest estimated nursing costs

- Total and average number of orders for parenteral infusions (per patient) in each unit for specific DRGs

- Total and average number of orders for vital signs evaluation (by unit and patient acuity level)

- Total and average number of orders for I&O level (by unit and patient acuity level)

- Total and average number of referrals for consultation with a clinical nurse specialist by:

  -type of clinical specialist
  -department/professional who made the request

- Utilization of the infection control practitioner by other nursing personnel based on:

  -number of referrals from nursing personnel to the infection control practitioner
  -attendance at educational programs given by the infection control practitioner
  -number of individual consultations between nursing personnel and the
   infection control practitioner

- Total number of referrals to outpatient nursing services/educational programs (by type of service and program)

- Total number of requests for nurses to perform non-nursing duties (by type of request: eg, physical therapy, respiratory therapy, housekeeping, transporting patients, etc)

- Total and average number of hours of nursing care (by payor category) for patients in specific age groups, such as:

  -0 - 17 years
  -18 - 40 years
  -41 - 65 years
  -66 - 80 years
  -over 80 years

- Total and average hours of nursing care (per patient) for the 10 highest-volume DRGs for the hospital

- Range of hours of nursing care (per patient) for the 25 highest-volume DRGs for the hospital

- Total and average hours of nursing care (per patient) for the 10 DRGs that have the highest total charges for the hospital

- Total and average hours of nursing care (per patient) for the 5 DRGs that have the highest estimated profit for the hospital

- Total projected relative value units (by type of procedure) for certain patient care procedures (eg, IV chemotherapy, tracheostomy care, admission assessment, peritoneal dialysis, etc)

- Total and average estimated nursing costs overall

- Total and average estimated nursing costs per patient in each unit

- Total and average estimated nursing costs for the 25 highest-volume DRGs for the hospital

- Total, range and average estimated nursing costs for the 10 DRGs that are ranked highest in terms of overall costs

- Distribution of discharges (by DRG) for each clinical unit

- Volume of discharged (by clinical unit) for the 25 highest-volume DRGs for the hospital

- Distribution of discharges (by DRG) for the 10 DRGs that have the highest estimated costs for the hospital, greatest use of overall hospital services and highest estimated costs for nursing services

- Distribution of discharges by type of discharge followup needed by patients, such as:

  -home health care
  -verbal/written reinforcement of activity restrictions
  -supportive equipment
  -continuing instruction

- Distribution of discharges of patients who have a chronic disease as the primary or secondary diagnosis by type of chronic disease (eg, diabetes mellitus, chronic obstructive lung disease, cardiovascular disease, etc)

Category I: Utilization Monitors

Subcategory B: Clinical Appropriateness and Timeliness of Admissions, Orders, and Referrals

Topics:

  - Appropriateness of admission of patients whose condition does not seem to warrant inpatient services

  - Appropriateness of admission of patients on Friday when no tests or therapies can be instituted until the following week (by physician and DRG)

  - Appropriateness of admission to a clinical unit based on patient's nursing and medical care needs

  - Appropriateness of placement of patients in clinical units based on staffing patterns and staff availability

  - Timeliness of patient transfers to general clinical units from admitting, the recovery room and other departments

  - Timeliness, completeness and legibility of information in physicians' progress notes that affect the nursing care needs of patients

- Timeliness of physicians' visits to patients who were admitted to clinical units directly from the recovery room after major, invasive procedures

- Timeliness of consultations for patients on general medical-surgical units who have psychiatric problems or who have abused drugs or alcohol

- Appropriateness of physicians' orders for medications to be left at the patient's bedside

- Appropriateness of physicians' orders for tests and procedures that could be done on an outpatient basis

- Apropriateness of repeat orders for tests, procedures and x-rays

- Appropriateness of diagnostic tests requested for patients in the three DRGs having the highest volume on a unit

- Appropriateness of IV therapy ordered for patients in a particular DRG or with a particular diagnosis (eg, diabetic acidosis)

- Appropriateness of physicians' standing orders

- Appropriateness/timeliness of orders for special therapies to be performed by nursing staff, specifically

  -ventilator-assisted respiration
  -renal dialysis
  -albumin infusions
  -transfusions of blood/blood products
  -TPN

- Timeliness with which therapies that are no longer required by the patient's condition have been discontinued, including

  -I & O measurements
  -vital signs readings
  -daily weights
  -traction
  -use of "K pads"
  -suction therapy
  -oxygen therapy
  -IPPB treatments

- Appropriateness of physician orders for new or experimental medications or treatments based on the current scope of nursing practice in the institution

- Appropriateness of nursing time spent in non-nursing functions such as

  -preparation of "piggyback" medications
  -passing and retrieving meal trays
  -transporting patients to other departments
  -"running" to pharmacy for medications

-relief of monitor clerk during breaks and the lunch hour
-relief of unit secretaries/ward clerks during breaks and the lunch hour

- Appropriateness of requests for nursing personnel to transfer patients within units or between units

- Delays in the timely discharge of patients due to lack of beds in extended care facilities/nursing homes

- Timeliness of physicians' orders for discharge planning, individual patient education or referral to outside agencies

- Timeliness of referrals to specialized nursing care or nurse specialists (eg, enterostomal care, diabetic education, clinical nurse specialist in cardiology, oncology, mental health)

- Timeliness of referrals to group educational programs sponsored by nursing (eg, diabetic classes, cardiac rehabilitation classes, stress management classes, etc)

- Appropriateness of nurses' standing orders or standardized nursing care plans

Category I: Utilization Monitors

Subcategory C: Clinicians' Use of Assessments and Recommendations Made by Staff Nurses, Clinical Nurse Specialists or Nurse Managers

Topics:

- Appropriate and timely use of nurses' preadmission assessment data in patient care planning

- Appropriate and timely use of nurses' admission assessments by physicians, nurses and social services to guide discharge planning

- Appropriate and timely use of information from nurses' admission assessment to guide other nurses in developing a nursing care plan*

  *NOTE: The phrase "nursing care plan" is used in its generic sense to denote a plan of care that focuses on the patient, his/her needs and health care problems and that is formulated jointly by the nurse, the patient and/or the family (significant others).

- Appropriate and timely use of the nursing care plan by nurses other than the primary nurse or the nurse who has initiated the plan

- Physicians' use of the nursing care plan to time patients' discharge

- Appropriate and timely use of nurse-to-nurse referrals between staff from inpatient care areas and staff in community agencies

- Appropriate and timely use of nurse-to-nurse referrals by staff in inpatient care areas

- Patients' use of information given by nurses in a specific educational program

- Patients' use of discharge information written by nursing personnel

Category II.   Departmental Performance Monitors

Subcategory A: Overall Departmental Performance Monitors

Topics:

- Mean nursing care hours produced per patient day

- Total and average number of nursing procedures performed by day, shift, month

- Total and average number of patients treated by day and month

- FTE: patient day ratio for the department

- Average patient caseload per nurse per shift

- Total and average hours of direct and indirect nursing care per patient for those 25 DRGs ranked highest by volume in the institution

- Total and average hours of direct and indirect nursing care per patient for those 10 DRGs having the highest volume for the nursing department

- Total and average hours of direct and indirect nursing care per patient for those five DRGs having the highest volume on each clinical unit

- Total and average number of admission assessments completed by the department

- Percentage of nursing care plans written for specific patient populations (by department and unit)

- Percentage of successful resuscitation (CPR) attempts

- Number of nursing personnel (by level) requested to take RIF (reduction in force) days weekly, monthly, quarterly

- Overtime hours paid to licensed and unlicensed nursing personnel by shift, unit, department

Category II.   Departmental Performance Monitors

Subgroup B: Performance of Specific Departmental Functions Involving Direct Patient Care

Topics:

1. Assessment Phase of the Nursing Process

   - Completeness of the assessment of the patient by an RN within a specified time of admission

- Completeness of the nursing assessment of the patient's condition on admission based on unit policy/procedures, medical diagnosis and patient care needs

- Appropriateness of nursing diagnoses based on patients' medical diagnosis/es

- Accuracy of nursing diagnoses based on the nursing assessment and nursing progress notes

- Inclusion of functional health pattern areas in the nursing assessment of patients, namely

   -health perception/health pattern management
   -nutritional/metabolic pattern
   -elimination pattern
   -activity/exercise pattern
   -sleep/rest pattern
   -cognitive/perceptual pattern
   -self-perception/self-concept pattern
   -role relationship pattern
   -sexuality/reproductive pattern

- Accuracy of assessment of patients' physical disabilities and/or need for prosthetic devices on admission (eg, contact lenses, dentures, hearing aids, etc)

- Appropriate and timely assessment of equipment needed for physical support of patients (eg, mattresses, pillows, splints, sand bags, trapeze, etc)

- Completeness of assessment of patients' mental/emotional state on admission and throughout their lengths of stay

- Timeliness of assessment of specified high-risk factors to identify patients who need discharge planning

- Appropriateness and timeliness of collaboration between nursing personnel and dietary personnel in the nutritional assessment of oncology patients

- Completeness of pain assessment for surgical/oncology or other patient population clusters

- Adequacy of postsurgical assessments of patients undergoing major surgery during the 12 hours after their return to the clinical unit

- Accuracy of identification of deviations in patient status from established physical/emotional norms

- Appropriate and timely recognition of signs and symptoms that require notification of the physician

- Incidence of failure of nursing personnel to assess important signs and symptoms associated with a specific patient condition

- Capability of nursing personnel to assess spiritual/religious needs of patients

- Appropriate and timely assessment of educational needs of patients who have a specific diagnosis, diagnostic procedure, condition (eg, aphasia) or requirement (eg, bedrest)

- Ability of nursing personnel to assess the patient's or family's need or readiness for learning

- Competence of nursing staff in interviewing/ communicating with patients and families (significant others)

2. Planning Phase of the Nursing Process

- Timeliness of completion of a written nursing care plan after admission of a patient

- Involvement of the patient, family members or significant others in the development of the nursing care plan

- Appropriateness of goals and actions in nursing care plans, given the patient's condition and expected length of stay

- Congruence between nursing diagnosis/es, nursing care plan objectives and nursing interventions ordered for the patient

- Ability of the nursing staff to establish appropriate patient care priorities in the nursing care plan

- Appropriate and timely integration of the medical care plan with the nursing care plan

- Appropriateness of the nursing care plan based on continued assessments

- Accuracy of nurses in designating patient care priorities in the nursing care plan

- Presence in the nursing care plan of nursing orders/ interventions for certain drug therapies, (eg, BP monitoring for patients on antihypertensives, I & O for patients on diuretics, etc)

- Inclusion in the nursing care plan of nursing interventions to reorient patients who have sensory deprivation, physiological imbalances, etc

- Inclusion in the nursing care plan of actions expected to be performed by the patient to enhance and maintain independence, given the patient's physical limitations

- Inclusion of orders in the nursing care plan for referrals of patients to appropriate community agencies/support groups postdischarge (eg, Reach to Recovery, Diabetes Association, etc)

- Appropriate and timely coordination by physicians and nurses in planning the discharge of patients

- Clarity of nursing orders in the nursing care plan (eg, specific activity, time frame and methods to carry out activity individualized to patients

3. Implementation Phase of the Nursing Process

- Accuracy of clinical decisions made by nursing personnel for patients with a specific diagnosis (eg, myocardial infarction, pulmonary edema, etc)

- Appropriateness of nursing interventions for a specific nursing diagnosis/deviation from established physical/emotional norms (eg, diminished sensory stimulation, sleep/rest deprivation)

- Adequacy of orientation of patients to the hospital environment during the admission process (eg, physical environment of room/unit, nurse call system, hospital routines such as meal times, visiting hours, etc)

- Adequacy of provisions for patients' physical privacy

- Adherence of nursing personnel to procedures for handling and safekeeping of patient's valuables

- Completeness and timeliness of personal hygiene measures given to patients (eg, mouth care, hair and nail care, skin care, etc)

- Timeliness of nurses' performance of procedures/therapies within established time frames (eg, hourly outputs, vital signs q2h, medications q6h, etc)

- Competence of nursing personnel on general care units in the performance of infrequently performed procedures, such as

   -application of traction (eg, Buck's, etc)
   -care of patients on special bed frames (eg, circle bed, wedge bed, etc)
   -assessment of patients with CNS pathology
   -application of leather restraints

- Adherence of nursing staff to written standards of care established by nursing department

- Accuracy of staff performance of procedures for taking lying/standing BP readings

- Accuracy of staff performance of Accucheck procedure for monitoring blood glucose

- Accuracy of nursing personnel in the performance of preps for radiology studies

- Accuracy of nursing personnel in the performance of preps for laboratory studies

- Compliance of nursing staff with procedures for maintaining IV therapy

- Compliance of nursing personnel to procedures for changing dressings over central lines

- Competence of nursing staff in the management of dialysis shunts

- Maintenance of patency of drainage tubes

- Maintenance of aseptic technique during procedures requiring sterility (eg, preparation of parenteral medications, dressing changes, etc)

- Competence of nursing personnel in the administration of mixed insulins

- Accuracy and timeliness of management of extravasation of chemotherapeutic agents by nursing personnel

- Compliance of nursing personnel to procedures for immobilizing injured extremities

- Compliance of nursing staff to procedures for positioning unconscious or comatose patients

- Accuracy of performance of nursing personnel during CPR codes

- Adherence of nursing personnel to procedures for designating and caring for "no code" patients

- Competence of nursing personnel in management of ventilator-assisted patients

- Turnaround time between the patient's call for assistance and response by nursing personnel

- Turnaround time between the patient's request for prn medication and the administration of medication by nursing personnel

- Productivity of shift overlap time for nurses working 10-hour shifts

- Capability of nursing personnel to give accurate, complete, timely, concise, pertinent information about patients in the shift report

- Provision of pertinent information by nursing staff to patients/family members (significant others) about the patient's condition and progress toward meeting the objectives of the nursing care plan

- Ability to counsel patients/families (significant others) in the development of effective coping skills related to

  -grief/loss
  -altered body image
  -dependency/independency conflict
  -sick role

- Competence of nursing personnel in conducting stress reduction activities for patients, family members (significant others)

- Appropriate use of patient educational materials that accommodate variations in culture, language, sensory impairments and educational levels

- Compliance of nursing personnel to policy regarding cancellation of preop medications at the time of patient surgery

- Compliance by nursing personnel to policy regarding automatic "stop" order guidelines on the administration of antibiotics

- Compliance by nursing personnel to policy to stop narcotics administration to patients after expiration date

- Incidents of insulin administration to diabetics who are NPO and have no glucose coverage

- Appropriate and timely coordination of patient therapy regimens between nursing and

  -pharmacy
  -physical therapy
  -occupational therapy
  -respiratory therapy
  -dietary

- Timeliness of coordination of respiratory treatments for patients who are receiving tube feedings

- Continuation of patient activities that support attainment of patients' physical therapy goals

- Quality of specimens obtained by nursing personnel for laboratory tests

- Completeness and accuracy of communication regarding patient treatments between nursing and

  -physical therapy
  -occupational therapy
  -respiratory therapy

- Timely and complete coordination of discharge planning/teaching among medical (or other professional) staff, nursing staff, patients and their families (significant others)

- Collaboration of physicians and nurses in completing discharge instruction forms

4. Evaluation Phase of the Nursing Process Related to Patient Outcomes

- Rate of achievement of goals stated in the nursing care plan for patients in specific DRGs or with specific nursing diagnoses

- Patient's achievement of specified or implied goals of therapy, such as

  -verbalization of feelings about dependency
  -weight loss
  -lowered blood pressure
  -self-care activities
  -adequate perfusion of tissues
  -adequate air exchange to allow for resumption of normal activities
  -stress reduction exercises during anxiety attacks

- Patient's level of knowledge of the role and accessibility of the patient representative/ombudsman

- Patient's ability to self-administer medications after instruction by nursing personnel

- Ability of cancer/ostomy patients to perform self-care following surgery and discharge after pre-operative teaching by nursing personnel

- Changes/differences in patient complication rates related to bedrest among different clinical units

- Changes/differences in lengths of stay of patients in the 25 DRGs having the highest volume in the institution (by unit)

- Complications of TPN therapy arising from failure to follow nursing protocols

- Degree of pain relief in patients following administration of pain relief measures by nursing staff

- Patients' understanding of the disease process, specifically the signs and symptoms that should be reported

- Patient/family awareness of the nursing care plan

- Patients' understanding of treatments/procedures occurring during hospitalization

- Patients' understanding of equipment that is being used during their therapy

- Patient/family knowledge of treatments that need to be performed postdischarge (eg, dressing changes, injection technique for medications, etc)

- Patients' understanding of medications for which they are responsible postdischarge (eg, name of medication, dosage, side effects, interaction with food and other drugs etc)

- Capability of oncology patients to perform self-care with Hickman catheters at time of discharge

- Adherence of patients to followup appointments in physicians' offices or outpatient departments or services

- Readmission of diabetic patients within 60 days of discharge

5. Evaluation Phase of the Nursing Process Related to Nursing Judgments that Affect Patient Outcomes

    - Timeliness of notification of the physician about a change in the patient's condition and/or the patient's concerns

    - Timeliness of notification of the physician about abnormal laboratory results

- Timeliness of response by nursing personnel to patients' critical conditions (eg, respiratory distress, hemorrhage, shock, cardiac arrhythmias, emotional crisis, etc)

- Timeliness of administration of prn medications, such as

  -sedatives
  -pain medications to surgical, oncology or other patient populations
  -antiemetics
  -antianxiety medications

- Appropriateness of the frequency of monitoring vital signs based on the patient's condition and the physician's orders

- Adequacy/timeliness of nursing interventions for patients suffering nausea and vomiting as a side effect of radiation or drug therapy

- Appropriateness/timeliness of nursing interventions to prevent constipation in elderly patients having barium studies

- Timeliness of nursing interventions for patients who are susceptible to or are experiencing nutritional deficiencies

- Appropriateness/timeliness of nursing interventions for patients suffering depression secondary to their physical illness

- Appropriateness/timeliness of referrals by nurses to other departments (eg, speech therapy, physical therapy, occupational therapy, social services, etc)

- Appropriateness of written discharge information given to patients

- Appropriateness/timeliness of submission of transfer information to the receiving facility/referral agency

Category II.   Departmental Performance Monitors

Subcategory C: Availability, Distribution and Appropriateness of Use of Departmental Resources

Topics:

1. Availability and Appropriateness of Staff Assignments

    - Staff: patient ratio on evening and night shifts and weekends (by unit)

    - Nursing staff: patient ratios by level of staff (eg, RN, LPN, aide)

    - Congruence between actual patient: staff ratios and the ratios suggested by patient classification data

    - Appropriateness of assignment of nursing personnel based on the nursing care needs of the patient, acuity data and institutional policies

- Stability of assignment of nursing personnel to the same patient group throughout the patient's length of stay

- Availability of nursing staff with specialized skills to provide therapy that has been ordered for patients (eg, chemotherapy)

- Availability of skilled nursing personnel to care for "off-service" patients who are placed on clinical specialty units

- Ability/availability of nursing personnel to be assigned to different units due to cross-training

- Availability of nursing personnel to cover sick time/vacation time by level of personnel (eg, RN, LPN, aide) and unit

- Availability of flexible (temporary) staff for call-in duty on days of higher-than-average acuity or census levels

- Availability of non-nursing personnel to assist with patient transfers on the general unit

- Appropriateness of utilization of LPNs for specialized procedures on units or in the department

- Utilization of float pool personnel and/or regular personnel to staff clinical units that need additional caregivers, including

  -number of personnel who are reassigned (by shift)
  -level of personnel being replaced
  -level of replacement personnel
  -units from which personnel are "pulled"
  -units to which additional personnel are assigned

- Percentage of nursing time spent in

  -direct patient care activities
  -specific nursing functions (eg, medication administration, patient assessment, basic hygiene measures, etc)
  -indirect patient care activities (eg, charting, care planning, order transcription, patient care conferences, etc)

- Nursing care time spent in duplicate charting of information

- Average number of telephone calls requiring nursing input (by unit and shift)

- Total and average time spent by nursing staff in patient teaching activities (per day, month)

- Total and average nursing staff time spent presenting educational programs (per month)

- Total and average time spent by nursing staff in individual consultation with other professionals

- Total and average nursing staff time spent at education programs (per month)

- Total and average time spent clarifying physicians' orders (per day, week, month)

- Total and average time spent in quality review activities per quarter (by level of personnel)

- Total and average time spent by professional staff in formal meetings (per week, month, quarter)

- Turnover rate of personnel per quarter (by level)

- Rate of absenteeism per employee (per quarter)

- Rate of tardiness per employee (per quarter)

- Average overtime hours paid per RN per year

- Average illness-related benefit hours paid per RN per year

2. Availability and Appropriateness of Equipment and Supply Allocations

- Turnover rate of stock supplies/medications on the clinical unit

- Availability of routine supplies on the exchange cart

- Availability of dietary stock items kept on patient care units

- Availability of functional equipment for direct patient care, specifically

    -IV pumps and poles
    -decubitus pads
    -wheelchairs
    -carts
    -sling scales/bed scales
    -trach adaptors for Ambubags
    -commodes
    -suction apparatus

- Availability of emergency equipment and supplies on the unit

- Availability of equipment needed to perform specific procedures on the unit (eg, cutdown trays, tracheostomy trays, thoracotomy trays, etc)

- Appropriateness and availability of materials used to give patients discharge instructions, namely

    -preps for post-discharge radiology studies
    -preps for post-discharge laboratory studies
    -medication information (eg, therapeutic effects, side effects, etc)

- Total downtime for the computer system in nursing care areas by day/week

- Cost of equipment and supplies by month/quarter, including

  -percentage of nursing budget allocated for equipment/supplies
  -costs of replacing equipment/supplies
  -costs of maintaining/stocking equipment/supplies
  -downtime for critical care equipment (eg, apnea monitors, cardiac monitors, ventilators, etc)

- Availability of private rooms/quiet rooms for patient and families (significant others) who require privacy

- Adequacy of clean linen supply on patient care units

Category II.   Departmental Performance Monitors

Subcategory D: Documentation

Topics:

1. Documentation Related to the Patient's Condition, Therapy and Progress

- Accuracy and completeness of documentation of medically prescribed treatment for a patient

- Discrepancies between physician's and nurses' progress notes

- Congruency between the level of acuity that has been assigned to patients by nursing personnel and documentation of acuity levels in medical records

- Total number of medical records with incomplete documentation of nursing care (per unit/department)

- Presence of judgmental, sarcastic or unprofessional notations in nurses' progress notes

- Legibility of nursing progress notes

- Accurate and timely completion of nursing assessment forms/nursing care plans by new orientees

- Accurate and timely completion of special chart forms by nursing personnel (eg, diabetic flow sheet, anticoagulant flow sheet, etc)

- Usefulness and clarity of format, number and kinds of chart forms for documenting patient care

- Completeness and timeliness of entries on preop checklists

- Accuracy and completeness of documentation of I&O measurements

- Accuracy, completeness and timeliness of documentation by nursing personnel of monitoring of patients in restraints

- Completeness, accuracy and timeliness of documentation of intravenous fluids administered to patients

- Accuracy, timeliness and completeness of documentation of tube feedings

- Accuracy and completeness of documentation of the patient's physical therapy done by nurses (eg, activity as ordered, tolerance to activity, degree of assistance needed by patient, etc)

- Completeness, accuracy and timeliness of documentation of medication administration to include

  -reasons why medications were not given
  -the patient's response to prn medications for pain, nausea, sedation, etc

- Completeness and timeliness of documentation of àdverse effects/complications of treatments given to patients

- Completeness and accuracy of nursing discharge notes at the time the patient is transferred from special care units

- Completeness and accuracy of documentation of health education efforts, including

  -knowledge gained by the patient/family (significant others)
  -behavioral changes made by the patient/family (significant others)
  -enhancement of patient/family (significant others) interaction with each other
   and with health team members

- Completeness and timeliness of documentation of diabetic patients' knowledge of self-care prior to discharge

- Completeness of discharge notes written by nursing personnel on the medical record

- Completeness and timeliness of documentation of referral instructions given to patients by nursing personnel

- Accessibility of the patient record to physicians, nurses and other health team members on the clinical unit

2. Documentation of Information Given to Patients and Agencies

- Completeness, accuracy and timeliness of transfer forms sent to hospitals within a metropolitan area

- Completeness and accuracy of written discharge information given to patients by nursing personnel

- Completeness and accuracy of transfer records sent to another facility/agency by nursing personnel

- Completeness and accuracy of information given on VNA referrals at the time of the patient's discharge

3. Documentation of Charge Information

- Completeness of information on charge slips

- Accuracy of the documentation of the charges for stock supplies or medications

- Accuracy of the documentation of the charges for supplies used from the exchange cart

- Accuracy of the documentation of the charges for fluids used in IV therapy

- Accuracy of the documentation of the charges for equipment (by type of item and by unit)

Category III: User Satisfaction Monitors

Topics:

- Patient's satisfaction with his/her orientation to the hospital at the time of admission

- Patient/family's (significant other's) perceptions regarding the courtesy shown by nursing personnel

- Patient's perception of the quality of communication with nursing personnel during their hospitalization

- Family's (significant other's) perception of the quality of nursing services provided to the patient

- Patient's satisfaction with the timeliness of the nursing staff's response to the call light

- Patient's satisfaction with the nursing staff's response to requests for pain relievers

- Patient's perception of the content, format and helpfullness of the group educational programs presented by nursing personnel

- Patient's satisfaction with individual teaching done by nursing personnel

- Patient's satisfaction with the quantity and quality of information provided by nursing personnel on self-care

- Patient/family's (significant other's) satisfaction with their ability to perform wound care following instruction by nursing personnel

- Patient's satisfaction with outpatient educational programs presented by nursing personnel (eg, stress management, management of diabetes, "geri-gym", etc)

- Patient's perception of his/her "perceived health status" on discharge as compared to his/her "perceived health status" on admission

- Patient's satisfaction with staff nurses' followup after discharge

- Physicians' satisfaction with the nursing care of their patients

- Physicians' satisfaction with individual consultations with nurses in planning patient care

- Physicians' satisfaction with the diabetic education program conducted by nursing personnel for their patients

- Nurses' satisfaction with pertinence and timeliness of consultations done by clinical nurse specialists

- Nurses' satisfaction with the appropriateness and timeliness of nurse-to-nurse consultations

- Hospital staff's perception of the competence of nursing personnel during cardiac arrest "codes"

- Billing/finance department's satisfaction with the accuracy/completeness of charge information submitted by nursing personnel

Category IV.   Safety Monitors

Topics:

- Performance of routine health checks of nursing personnel (eg, TB tests)

- Frequency and amount of exposure of nursing personnel to cytotoxic agents

- Rate of hepatitis-B vaccination among employees who work in high-risk areas

- Staff knowledge of potential safety hazards associated with unit equipment

- Accuracy and timeliness of staff response to fire/disaster drills

- Adherence to written standards of care for treating patients who are at high-risk for falls

- Appropriateness of use of siderails for specific patient populations (eg, elderly, comatose, etc)

- Adherence to departmental procedures for handwashing

- Timeliness of handwashing of nursing personnel

- Appropriateness and timeliness of placement of patients who have infectious diseases

- Appropriateness and timeliness of placement of patients who have increased susceptibility to infection

- Adherence to isolation procedures (eg, respiratory, wound and skin, etc) for patients with specific types of infection

- Adherence to precautions when treating patients who receive oxygen

Category V: Quality Control Monitors

Topics:

1. Attainment and Maintenance of Skill Levels

    - Verification of current licensure of all RNs and LPNs

    - Verification of yearly BCLS certification of all nursing staff

    - Verification that nurses have the skills necessary to treat patients in a particular unit or specialty area or to perform specific procedures

    - Verification that float staff have specialized skills for treating patients in special care units or the pediatric or OB areas

    - Completeness and timeliness of documentation of nursing skills during staff orientation to the institution/unit

    - Maintenance of updated skills inventory on all nursing staff on a clinical unit

    - Timeliness of required performance appraisals of staff on each unit

    - Timeliness of performance appraisals of new orientees on each unit

    - Accuracy of orders transcribed by nursing personnel

    - Adherence to procedures for handling controlled substances

    - Security of maintenance of/access to "narcotic" keys (by shift and unit)

    - Appropriateness/adequacy of continuing education programs attended by nursing personnel

    - Review/revision of policies and procedures related to direct patient care on each unit and for the entire department

2. Quality of Equipment and Supplies

    - Adequacy of ventilation, humidification and/or temperature control of patients' rooms

    - Conditions of brakes on beds, stretchers and wheel chairs in each unit and the entire department

    - Timeliness of scheduled maintenance checks on monitors and emergency equipment.

    - Thoroughness of crash cart checks (per shift/day)

    - Timeliness of staff reporting of faulty or inoperative equipment

Category VI.   Incident/Occurrence Monitors

Topics:

- Deaths within 24 hours of admission

- Deaths with 24 hours of discharge

- Unplanned admissions to critical care units

- Unplanned transfers to other hospitals

- Readmission of patients within 60 days of discharge for treatment of complications related to the previous hospitalization

- Rate of unintended adverse outcomes of procedures or treatments by type (eg, infiltration of IVs, diarrhea associated with tube feedings, etc)

- Complications/adverse reactions to specific treatments or medications (eg, burns due to heat lamps, phlebitis due to IV therapy, etc) among patients

- Number of delayed nursing diagnoses that resulted in a complication

- Clarity/adequacy of designation of "no code" orders for terminal patients

- Complications due to trauma during CPR (eg, fractured ribs, pneumothorax, lacerated liver, etc)

- Falls in each unit and the entire department (by age group, DRG, acuity level)

- Rate of nosocomial infections (by unit, physician, DRG)

- Rates of urinary tract infection among patients who have indwelling catheters

- Complications among patients who receive blood products (by unit)

- Incorrect intravenous infusions by type of error (too fast or too slow and patient diagnosis)

- Decubitus ulcer formation in each unit and the entire department

- Failure of nursing personnel to notify the physician of a significant change in patient status

- Number of times medications, treatments, tests or procedures have been mistakenly omitted

- Performance of procedures outside the scope of practice of nursing personnel (eg, a nursing assistant monitoring IV therapy)

- Adherence to protocols for managing emergency situations (eg, hemorrhage, cardiac arrest, respiratory arrest, shock, etc)

- Medication errors in each unit and the entire department

- Distribution of medication errors in each unit and the entire department by type of drug

- Breaches of procedure for handling controlled substances

- Administration of drugs to patients after their "stop-order" (expiration) date, especially for

  -antibiotics
  -narcotics

- Discharges of patients who do not meet nursing criteria for discharge (by unit, service and physician)

- Total and average number of discharges against medical advice (by unit and diagnostic category)

- Timeliness of notification of supervisor of discharges against medical advice

- Absence of appropriate written consent forms on the medical record

- Breaches of confidentiality of patient information by nurses

- Inaccurate transcription of physicians' orders for medications or inconsistencies between medication sheets and the medication Kardex file

- Number of times patients' valuables have been damaged or lost

- Number of complaints from patients/families about nursing services rendered (by unit)

- Rate of employee injuries in each unit and the entire department (by type of injury)

- Number and dollar amounts of workers' compensation claims submitted by nursing personnel in each unit and for overall department (by type of claim)

Category VII.   Monitors of Patient Management and Clinical Practices of Other Departments

Topics:

- Timeliness of delivery of "old charts" from the medical record department to the clinical unit

- Timeliness of administration of STAT, preliminary and initial doses of medication (by shift and unit)

- Number of "missing medications" on unit dose cart from pharmacy (by type of drug and unit)

- Turnaround time of STAT orders for laboratory tests, drugs or radiology tests or procedures

- Turnaround time for posting alert values by the laboratory

- Timeliness of dietary services given to patients at times other than scheduled meal times

- Timeliness of transfers of patients to and from the clinical unit and other departments for surgery, tests, procedures or therapy

- Availability of equipment in other departments to support patient care needs while patients are undergoing tests, procedures or other therapy (eg, suction equipment in physical therapy for patients with tracheostomies)

- Competence of staff in other departments to continue patient care therapies while patients are undergoing tests, procedures or other therapies (eg, capability of radiology staff to maintain an IV)

- Coordination of treatment based on the attending physician's orders and consulting professionals' recommendations

- Timeliness of response of other departments to referrals by nursing personnel, including

  - speech therapy
  - physical therapy
  - social services
  - occupational therapy
  - dietary services
  - respiratory therapy

- Rate of turnaround time for beds after patients have been transferred/discharged, especially "STAT" beds in special care units

- Timeliness of the scheduling sequence for diagnostic x-rays

- Orders for cephalosporins for patients who have not had C & S or whose C & S report indicates a low cost drug would be effective

- Incidence of headaches among patients who have had a myelogram and CT scan on the same day

- Degree of cleanliness of the unit kitchen, medication rooms maintained by the housekeeping department

- Degree of cleanliness of patient care areas (including patient rooms, visitor lounges, examination rooms, etc) maintained by the housekeeping department

- Appropriateness of diets and refreshments served to patients

7: Choosing High-Priority Topics

The number and variety of monitoring topics from which nurse managers can develop a comprehensive monitoring program can be overwhelming. In addition to topics that are currently included in the department's monitoring effort, nurse managers may create an extensive list of topics they *wish* they could monitor this list may include topics that were:

- Suggested in Chapter 6 for each category and subcategory of monitors

- Requested by nursing personnel, including nursing staff and the nursing administration

- Requested by members of other departments, the hospital administration and/or the medical staff

Monitoring the topics on a lengthy "wish list" will likely exceed available resources, support, staff and time. Therefore, nurse managers must cull, from the lists of actual and potential monitoring topics on the Unit/Department Monitoring Profile, the topics that will be of most value to them, their staff and the hospital administration.

Selecting High-Priority Monitoring Topics

Nurse managers in collaboration with departmental and hospital-wide QA professionals, should select from the Unit/Department Monitoring Profile only those topics that have high priority. High-priority topics are those that will generate the information the hospital and the department most urgently need to measure quality, efficiency and cost. As priority items, these monitors should be placed at the top of the department's monitoring schedule for the next six or twelve months, and they should be considered intrinsic parts of the work plan of the department.

Scanning Monitors

The following guidelines can be used to select high-priority SCANNING MONITORS from the Monitoring Profile:

1. Choose at least one topic in each of the seven categories:

   Utilization, Departmental Performance, User Satisfaction, Safety, Quality Control, Incident/Occurrence, and Patient Management and Clinical Practices of Other Departments.

2. For each category, choose topics that are believed to be the best barometers of departmental functioning or clinical practice. These topics describe problems that simultaneously affect the efficiency of operations and the quality of services. For example:

   - Availability of nursing staff with specialized skills to provide specific therapies that have been ordered for patients (eg, streptokinase drips, intraaortic balloon pump, ventilators, CVP, etc)

   - Timeliness of referrals to nurses who provide specialized care (eg, enterostomal therapists, diabetic educators, clinical nurse specialists in cardiology, oncology, mental health, etc)

   - Appropriateness of standing nursing orders in the unit and the department standards of nursing care and standardized nursing care plans

   - Assessment by nursing personnel of high-risk factors to identify patients who need discharge planning

   - Performance by nursing personnel of inadequate or inappropriate preps for tests or procedures to be done by staff in other departments

   - Availability of properly functioning equipment for direct patient care (eg, IV pumps, wheelchairs, sling/bed scales, suction apparatus, etc)

3. Choose topics required by the JCAH, AOA and regulatory organizations. These topics will fall under the categories of Departmental Performance, Safety, Quality Control and Incident/Occurrence Monitors.

   Many JCAH and AOA standards or governmental or licensing regulations can serve as topics of SCANNING MONITORS. For example:

   - Assessment of patients by an RN on admission to the institution

   - Presence of a written nursing care plan for patients within 24 hours of admission

   - Appropriateness of assignment of nursing personnel based on the nursing care needs of the patient and data from the patient classification system

   - Accuracy and completeness of documentation of prescribed treatments performed by nursing personnel for a patient

- Response of nursing personnel to fire/disaster drills

- Timeliness of routine health checks of nursing personnel (eg, TB tests)

- Verification of current licensure of all RNs and LPNs

- Verification of yearly BCLS certification of all nursing staff

- Verification of staff nurses skills during orientation to the institution or unit

4. Choose topics that will track changes in the delivery of hospital or nursing services that may result from cost-containment efforts.

   a. Some topics can measure the access to care for certain patient groups. Topics may include:

   - Distribution of patient admissions by payor status

   - Length of stay of patients by payor status

   - Nursing care hours per patient day by payor status

   - Availability of various services/facilities (eg, diabetic classes, cardiac rehabilitation classes) by payor category

   - Timeliness of response by nursing personnel to patients' requests for pain medication by specific patient populations, such as:

     -patients over 80 years of age

     -patients on Medicaid

     -patients with a specific ethnic background

   b. Certain topics can identify admissions that have been delayed too long, such as:

   - Average acuity level of patients (by day of stay) for selected DRGs

   - Morbidity/mortality rates of patients for selected DRGs

   c. Certain topics can monitor discharges that are occurring too early, such as:

   - Rate of readmission of patients within 30 days of discharge

   - Readmission of patients to treat complications related to a previous admission

   - Discharge of patients prior to the accomplishment of the goals/objectives listed in the nursing care plan

   - Degree to which physicians use the nursing care plan to time the discharge of patients

   - Type of discharge followup needed by patients, including

     -home health care

     -verbal/written reinforcement of activity restrictions

-supportive equipment

-continuing instruction

5. Choose topics that will provide information on how to increase the profitability or marketability of departmental services.

Examples

- The director of nursing medical/surgical care units collaborated with the director of pharmacy in one hospital to monitor the types of patients who receive long-term antibiotic therapy or TPN and determine how many patients could be treated effectively in a home therapy program. They decided to gather the information for one quarter and, if there were a sufficient number of cases, to project the costs of providing antibiotics or TPN to patients at home. They planned to compare the costs of home therapy to the current costs of hospitalization and ascertain whether a home antibiotic/TPN program would reduce costs for nursing services and the pharmacy and therefore result in cost savings for the patient and the institution.

- The director of nursing services in one hospital found that admissions and lengths of stay of patients with diabetes mellitus were dropping substantially. From previous monitoring efforts, the director knew that the department had a set of teaching materials for diabetic patients that facilitated learning and a core of staff nurses who were experienced in the teaching of diabetics. Because of the shortened lengths of stay of diabetic patients, however, the director of nursing services believed patients' educational needs were not being met in the inpatient setting. She therefore instituted a monitor of the learning needs of diabetics who had been discharged from the institution during one quarter to identify needs that were not being met and planned to use the information to justify a diabetic teaching program in an outpatient setting.

Focused Monitors

These guidelines can be used to select high-priority FOCUSED MONITORS from the Monitoring Profile.

1. Choose topics involving problems that immediately imperil the accreditation or licensing status of the hospital or the department. Deficiencies in the following areas of nursing operations provide examples of some of the types of problems that threaten accreditation or licensure:

- Nursing staff's adherence to procedures for handling controlled substances

- Nursing staff's maintenance of crash cart checks during each shift/day

- Staff compliance to isolation procedures (eg, respiratory, enteric, wound, etc) for patients who have specific types of infection

- Accuracy/completeness of documentation by nursing personnel concerning the administration of routine medications

- Presence of realistic and measurable goals in the nursing care plan, given the patient's condition and anticipated length of stay

2. Choose topics involving problems related to patient outcomes.

- Capability of parents upon discharge of infant from neonatal special care unit to use monitoring equipment and interpret monitoring data

- Effectiveness of nursing interventions to obtain pain control in children

- Appropriateness of nurses' triage decisions in the emergency department

- Appropriateness and timeliness of nurses' management of patients who have known or suspected contagion

- Rate of falls per unit (by patient age group and acuity level)

- Rate of complications among patients who receive blood products

- Failure of nursing personnel to notify the physician about a significant change in the patient's status

3. Choose topics that will provide objective evidence to administration that the quality of nursing services has been seriously impeded by recent cost-cutting measures.

Examples

- Cutbacks of staff in one nursing services department were made because the census had diminished over the past two years. Although the associate administrator for nursing agreed that staff cutbacks were necessary, she pointed out that while the census was dropping, the acuity level of patients was increasing markedly. The associate administrator therefore recommended that fewer staff cutbacks be made and that reductions be restricted to nonprofessional nursing personnel. However, the executive board of the hospital, believing that the reliability of the patient acuity data had not been adequately established, voted for full, across-the-board staff reductions. The associate administrator in nursing immediately instituted monitors to track the effects of the cutbacks. These monitors included:

- Incidence of unwitnessed cardiac arrests

- Incidence of patients' self-extubation

- Rates of decubitus ulcer formation in each unit

- Number and type of procedures ordered by physicians or nurses that were not performed by nursing staff

- Number of complaints from patients, families and physicians about the quality of nursing services

- The materials management department in one institution purchased a cheaper urinary catheterization kit despite concerns expressed by the nursing staff in a pilot study. Because the kit was difficult to open, its contents were frequently contaminated, and several kits had to be used for one procedure. The quality assurance committee in nursing monitored the actual cost of using the new kits and their impact on the quality of patient care. Through this effort, the committee demonstrated that the "cheaper kits" were costlier to the institution than the previous ones had been. The committee found that (1) more new kits had to be used, which raised the overall cost of catheterizations, (2) the kits were associated with a high incidence of urinary tract infections, which raised the cost of patient care.

- The vice-president of nursing services in one hospital felt that having an enterostomal therapist on staff was "nice" but not essential. She felt that staff nurses could provide the service just as well as the therapist could—and at less cost. Believing that the enterostomal therapist may actually be less costly to the institution, a group of nurse managers began to monitor:

  - Number of patient contacts made by the therapist

  - Services rendered during each contact with a patient

  - Patient, family and physician satisfaction with the therapist's services

  - Length of stay of patients who received the therapist's services

  - Length of stay of patients who did not receive the therapist's services but had a condition or underwent surgery that often requires enterostomal care

  With these data, the nurse managers planned to compute:

  - Costs of the inservices that would be needed to prepare staff nurses to assume the scope of services provided by the enterostomal therapist

  - Nursing care time and nursing cost per patient for enterostomal care performed by the therapist

  - Projected nursing care time and nursing cost per patient for enterostomal care performed by staff nurses

  - Difference in length of stay for patients who received the therapist's services and the length of stay for those who did not

  The managers thereby hoped to demonstrate the cost benefit of having the enterostomal therapist on staff.

4. Choose topics that will provide objective evidence requested by clinical committees and administration concerning inappropriate use of resources by physicians or nurses.

   Examples of such topics may include:

   - Admissions of patients whose condition does not seem to warrant inpatient services

   - Appropriateness of orders for portable chest x-rays of patients on general care units

- Requests by nursing personnel for STAT laboratory tests that have not been designated as STAT tests by the physician

- Referral of patients for discharge planning who do not meet the criteria for referral

5. Choose topics for which data are most accessible and with which significant problems may be detected.

Examples

- While tracking the changes in demographics for hospitalized patients over the last two years, the director of nursing services noticed a 50% increase in admissions of patients over age 75. Since the risk management department kept specific statistics on the incidence of falls in the institution, the nurse managers of the general care units felt they could quickly determine if the current "falls reduction program" was meeting the needs of the hospital's increasingly more elderly patient population. The nurse managers therefore worked with the risk management department to monitor the incidence of falls among patients over age 75.

- The head nurse of the pediatrics unit in one institution was able to update the standards of care of patients who have IV infusions by gathering information from several sources. The head nurse:

  -asked the infection control nurse to forward for the next quarter statistics on the incidence of phlebitis and infection associated with IV infusions in her unit

  -asked the quality assurance coordinator in nursing to forward for the next quarter the information she continuously collected on the number and cause of errors involving IV solutions in pediatrics

  -arranged for medical records personnel to collect data on the completeness of nursing documentation of IV therapy for patients discharged from the pediatrics unit within the next quarter

  -worked with the QA team on her unit to monitor the initiation and maintenance of IV infusions by nursing staff

  By summarizing the information from these multiple sources, the head nurse was confident that she could evaluate the quality with which IV infusions were currently being managed by nursing personnel, identify any problems in management and update departmental procedures for performing this treatment modality.

- During an accreditation visit to one hospital, a JCAH surveyor noted that documentation of the administration of routine medications was consistently incomplete on three clinical units. Shortly afterward, the hospital instituted a computerized system of charting the administration of medications that identified and reported any omissions in documentation. For the next two quarters, the head nurses on the clinical units that had been cited by the surveyor scanned daily computerized reports of omissions in charting routine medications and immediately followedup on them. Over the two quarters of the monitoring, the head nurses noted continual improvement. They consequently stopped reviewing daily computerized reports at the end of the monitoring period.

Summary

The selection of high priority topics for the monitoring program in nursing is a critical component of planning an agenda of QA monitors. No nursing unit or department has the resources—staff, time or money—to tackle an entire "wish list" of monitors. Nurse managers should collaborate with nursing staff and QA professionals to select only those monitors that have a high priority. Guidelines to facilitate selection of high priority monitors were presented in this chapter.

Once the topics for monitoring have been chosen, full specifications for each monitor must be developed. Guidelines for developing these specifications are discussed in the next chapter.

8: Completing the Specifications for Monitors

After selecting high priority topics, nurse managers must take one more step before they can begin to institute a departmental monitoring program. They must write "specs" or specifications for the monitoring topics they have chosen to describe how each monitor will be structured. Specifications must be written to describe the:

- Data to be collected

- Sources from which to collect the data

- Frequency and amount of data that should be collected

- Content and frequency of summary reports

- Duration of the monitor, including when it should be started, stopped and/or reappraised

- Name of the person(s) to collect and summarize data

- Criteria or goal statements that will be used to evaluate summary reports

- Sources of the criteria

Data to be Collected

Principle: Whenever possible, data collection needs should be stated in such a way that the actual collection of the data can be delegated to someone other than the department manager or a member of the nursing staff, preferably to a clerical person.

When specifying the data to be collected, the nurse manager must itemize the precise events, items and variables that should be counted or measured on a repeated basis. For most topics, data will have to be collected on the frequency with which something does or does not occur. And in order to make comparisons, information about several items will have to be collected for each monitor. For example, when monitoring staff performance of procedures within established time frames, the data to be collected will include the name of the procedure, the frequency with which it was ordered (ie, qh, 12h) and the frequency with which it was performed.

In general, data from SCANNING MONITORS will involve the frequency of the events, items or variables that are being measured. Consequently, data can be collected by clerical personnel or can be summarized from information in computer information systems.

Data from FOCUSED MONITORS, on the other hand, commonly concern clinical aspects of the department's functioning. Often, the data are related to appropriate clinical use of departmental services and will require review of individual patient records to determine whether the patient's signs and symptoms, test results or other clinical information justify use of the services. In such cases, data will be collected by the QA or UR coordinator or nursing personnel using criteria established by nursing staff or managers. In other circumstances, the data to be collected will specify the patterns of practice that warrant further analysis by a committee.

Example

If the UR coordinator or someone else with clinical knowledge and access to patient records is monitoring the appropriateness of vital signs evaluation, he or she may request data to be collected on:

- The number of orders (by nurses or physicians) for vital signs evaluation to be done more than once a day

- The acuity level and day of stay of each patient who has vital signs evaluation more than once a day

On the other hand, collection of these data is not the most efficient way to monitor the use of vital signs evaluation. Since the purpose of the monitor is to identify any unnecessary use of vital signs evaluation, the data collection task would be done more efficiently if it focused on the circumstances that warrant further investigation. For example, the UR coordinator may wish to collect data on the number of orders for vital signs evaluation to be done more than once a day when:

- The patient is being discharged that day

- The patient's acuity level is 1

- Vital signs have been within normal ranges for two days

These data can be used by the professional practice committee in nursing to determine when vital signs evaluation was appropriate during a review of the patient's medical records.

Data Sources

Principles: The choice of data sources must balance two considerations:

1. Ease of data collection from the data source

2. Accuracy of the data source

    Data sources for SCANNING MONITORS should be chosen on the basis of the ease of data collection. Data sources for FOCUSED MONITORS should be chosen on the basis of accuracy.

Working in collaboration with nursing staff, QA and UR professionals, data processing personnel, the manager of the medical record department and other members of the administration, managers in nursing services should determine the kinds of data that are available inside and outside the department. Such collaboration will help determine the:

- Assistance that realistically can be expected from current or projected hospital-wide information systems

- Assistance that will be available from QA and UR personnel

- Extent to which data collection can rely on existing data sources in the department

- Extent to which data collection will require department staff to create new data sources and/or collect data manually

To make the most efficient use of the manager's time and the department's and the hospital's resources, existing data sources should be used as much as possible. Hospital data sources and data sources routinely maintained in the department frequently provide all the information that is needed for a monitor. Hospital data sources that are available to department managers include:

- Patient satisfaction surveys

- Incident reports

- Infection control data

- Credentialing reviews

- Case-mix reports

- Financial reports

- Patients' bills

- Logs maintained by other departments and personnel

Manual and automated data sources that are maintained in a department include:

- Departmental logs

- Copies of orders for and reports of completed clinical studies

- Copies of orders for medications

- Quality control checks

- Findings from prospective, concurrent and retrospective review studies

- Staffing schedules

- Budgets

- Management reports

Sometimes, data for a monitor can be pulled together from several hospital and departmental documents, such as:

- Reports documenting the lack of availability of emergency equipment or drugs hospitalwide and check lists from departmental crash cart checks

- Results of patient questionnaires on the timeliness of nurses' response to requests for assistance during off shifts and weekends and the staffing schedules for those specific times

- The acuity report and schedule of nursing personnel for each unit

- Number of charges for IV solutions submitted by nursing personnel and pharmacy reports of the number of IV solutions dispensed to clinical units

Data for some monitors may be obtained from the patient's medical record and a hospital or departmental document. Examples of such instances may include:

- Patient bills showing charges for medications and medication records on patients' charts

- Hospital incident reports on the loss of patient valuables and admission sheets documenting patients' valuables

- Phlebitis rates associated with IV therapy and documentation of IV therapy in nurses' progress notes

Other monitors will require screening of patients' records exclusively. Screening is necessary when data must be gathered on patients' signs and symptoms or their response to treatment. Occasionally, new sources of data will have to be created for monitors that involve observing staff performance, conducting surveys or maintaining special logs for short periods.

If existing hospital and department data sources cannot meet the data collection needs for a monitor, the nurse manager should weigh the advantages and disadvantages of using other data sources and data collection methods. He/she should decide which:

- Source will yield data in the most useful form

- Source will provide the most accurate data

- Method of data collection will interfere the least with the time and responsibilities of involved staff

- Method of data collection will cost the least

The advantages and disadvantages of six data sources and data collection methods are summarized on pages 112 and 113.

Frequency and Amount of Data Collection

Principles: Enough data should be collected so the nurse manager will feel confident about making estimates and drawing conclusions from summary reports. The amount of data should not exceed what can be collected and analyzed efficiently within the context of the staff's usual activities.

Two of the most difficult decisions to make about a monitor are how much and how frequently data should be collected. Making these determinations is as much an art as it is a science because nurse managers cannot fall back on a set number of cases for a set period of time for every monitor. Monitors, as defined in Chapter 1, are mechanisms for the repeated collection of data. "Repeated" does not mean that data must be collected on every single case, every single day—forever! But how can nurse managers choose the number of cases to be reviewed?

DATA COLLECTION METHODOLOGIES

Method	Advantages	Disadvantages
Use of information from existing hospital records	Record-keeping procedures need not be changed. Records may be easily obtained. It is inexpensive.	The information must be taken as given, and it may not be organized in the proper form.
Review of patient records	The method provides objective clinical information. Reviewers easily identify samples within patient populations.	The process is time-consuming and costly if large numbers of records must be reviewed. Patient records cannot always provide the necessary information.
Observation	A disinterested (objective) individual who is not involved in the activity under study or a videotape monitor collects the data. Actual nursing care delivered to patients can be assessed. The observer also can provide narrative comments on what is being observed.	The process is expensive and time-consuming. Staff members feel they are "being watched."
Written surveys	Surveys collect information, particularly subjective views, that is not possible otherwise. Surveyors control the sample.	Questionnaires are difficult to design and time-consuming to use. It is often difficult to get complete and accurate responses to survey questions. There is a bias toward those who are willing and able to fill out the questionnaires.

DATA COLLECTION METHODOLOGIES (Continued)

Method	Advantages	Disadvantages
Interviews	Interviews personalize the observation technique. Interviewers can probe issues deeply and obtain followup on certain key points.	The process is very time-consuming. Creating a standard approach with several interviewers is difficult. Subjectivity is difficult to eliminate. Interviews usually interrupt or interfere with staff members' customary duties.
Compiling logs	The method provides current information about a monitor. The method collects data that may be used in several different ways (eg, for calculating demand for a procedure, the time needed to perform the procedure, cost of supplies for that procedure, etc).	Compiling logs is time-consuming for staff. Logs often are kept erratically. Some staff may feel they have to make themselves "look good" and record what they think the manager wants instead of what actually happens.

Formal statistical methods explain how to make estimates about a sample's size with confidence. However, these methods are often complex, and they are most useful for formal research. For monitoring purposes, some simple benchmarks can be used. The simplest is for the nurse manager to use his/her or the staff's knowledge of the topic as a guide. As a general rule, the *less that is known* about a topic, the *more cases* that must be included in the sample.

Another simple benchmark involves the scope of the topic. The *greater the volume* of patients, orders or studies for a particular topic, the *more cases* that must be reviewed. But the *more focused* or *homogeneous* the involved group or procedure, the *fewer cases* that need to be studied.

The department manager has two options:

Option 1:   Review all cases

This approach can be followed when:

- Data are available on an automated system and summary data can be amassed easily

- Very few cases or situations occur

- The adverse affect on patients, visitors or staff is so severe that every occurrence should be reviewed (absolute frequency)

- A situation occurs during a brief period of time, such as between 3 PM and 4 PM

Option 2:   Review a sample of available cases

A sample of available cases should be taken when:

- Absolute frequency does not have to be determined

- A large number of cases is available

- The situation is widespread among staff and/or patients

- The group in the sample is homogeneous (eg, patients with diabetes mellitus who have been diagnosed in the last six months)

When choosing a sample, the nurse manager may:

a.   Restrict the sample to a specific time period and repeat the sample periodically, for example:

-all cases during the last week of every month

-all cases in January, March, May and July

b. Establish a fixed quantity of cases to evaluate regardless of time period and screen cases until the number is reached, for example:

-ten cases per month for which a patient referral was made by a nurse to another hospital department

-three cases per nurse for a specific procedure

-the next 50 medication errors in special care units

c. Combine the two, for example:

-a sample of 50 cases every three months

Frequency and Content of Summary Reports

Principles: The frequency with which data should be summarized depends on the amount of data gathered during the time period in question. Large numbers of cases or situations should be summarized more frequently than small numbers. Monthly summaries will be needed in some instances, but quarterly summaries are sufficient for most monitors. Data should be summarized at least semiannually.

Summary reports should show both the total and the average figures for the time period in question and the cumulative total and average for the entire monitoring period.

In most cases, the summary reports for a monitor will match the manner in which data were requested. For example, if a monitor of unplanned admissions of patients from general care units to special care units collected data on the:

- Number of unplanned admissions during the reporting period by unit, physician and patient diagnosis

- Number and type of special procedures/treatments initiated on the day the patient was admitted to the special care unit

The summary report would show the:

- Total number of unplanned admissions for each unit, physician and patient diagnosis during the reporting period

- Total number and percent distribution of special procedures/treatments initiated on the day of the patient's admission to the special care unit

In addition to the total and average figures, some summary reports will show the "rate" or percentage of time that something occurred. For example, if a monitor collected the following information:

- Number of FTE days scheduled for each clinical unit

- Number of absentee/sick days for each clinical unit

The summary report would show:

$$\frac{\text{number of absentee/sick days}}{\text{number of FTE days scheduled}} \times 100 = \text{Rate of absenteeism}$$

Summary reports may contain incidental information that was collected in conjunction with the monitor, such as problems with documentation or other problems encountered in conducting the monitor.

Duration of the Monitor

Principles: The duration of a monitor depends on its nature. Monitors required by regulatory agencies or monitors of high-risk procedures or topics should be conducted at least once a year. Monitors that disclose problems or show that the department is not meeting expected goals should be continued until the problem is corrected or the goals are met. All monitors should be reappraised at least once a year to determine whether different or additional data should be collected and whether the monitor should be discontinued or conducted with more or less frequency.

SCANNING MONITORS of departmental functioning and performance are usually planned for one year before they are reappraised. FOCUSED MONITORS should be planned on a quarterly basis. SCANNING and FOCUSED MONITORS of topics that are required by regulatory agencies should be conducted as specified in the regulations.

SCANNING and FOCUSED MONITORS of patient care procedures that have significant adverse effect on patients if expectations are not met should be conducted continuously. However, if no problems are revealed in the first year of monitoring, data may be collected only once or twice in the following years to ensure that the department is meeting the expected level of achievement. When reappraising a monitor, the nurse manager should consider the following questions:

- Is the information provided by the monitor useful?

- Does the information provided by the monitor justify the time spent in data collection?

- Can the amount of data be reduced?

- Are additional data needed to "make sense" of the results of the monitor?

- Is the same information available in another way from other reports?

- Can the same information or almost the same information be obtained more easily?

- Are the data being summarized in too much or too little detail?

- Should the criteria that are used to evaluate summary data be modified?

- Should the same or different people collect the data?

- Has the monitor revealed any problems? Have steps been taken to correct the problems?

- Should the monitor be continued at least for a short period of time or periodically repeated to ensure that a problem that has been corrected does not recur?

Person to Collect and Summarize Data

Principle: Data collection should be assigned to a staff member who works with the data source as part of his/her usual responsibilities, and whenever appropriate and possible, it should be assigned to a nonprofessional person.

For many monitors, especially SCANNING MONITORS, data collection will be done automatically as part of an existing, automated information management system, such as patient accounts, case-mix data or departmental information systems. Data collection for other monitors may be done by someone outside the department who is already scrutinizing the quality and efficiency of services. In many hospitals, the QA, UR and/or DRG coordinators conduct limited data collection for department managers. Nurse managers should learn in advance the extent to which personnel outside the department will be available to help collect and summarize monitoring data.

The nurse manager should not attempt to personally collect all the data that are not available in automated systems or collected by outside personnel. The nurse manager should analyze the data collection requirements for each monitor and assign responsibility to the staff person who can collect the data most easily and/or most cost-effectively. Answers to the following questions will help the nurse manager choose the best person to collect and summarize data:

- Does the person have to know nursing/medical/technical terminology?

- Does the person have to be able to interpret technical and/or clinical information related to the monitor?

- To what extent must the person have personal contact with patients or others who use the department's services?

- Can the events, items and variables be defined clearly enough so a non-professional can collect the data?

- Must the person have access to patient records?

Criteria Used to Evaluate Summary Data and Initiate Further Investigation and Criteria Sources

Principles: A criterion, expectation or goal states the level of achievement that should be reflected in the summary data. Criteria should be written on the assumption that nonprofessional personnel will be collecting and summarizing the data. Criteria should specify precisely what aspects of summary data demonstrate that performance is at an acceptable level: the numbers, rates or other statistics that indicate adequate performance. Criteria also should specify when a professional needs to review the cases, items or events: the numbers, rates or other statistics that indicate levels of achievement were not met.

This is the most difficult part of writing specifications for a monitor because nurse managers must state in advance what will and what will not be acceptable to them. Criteria are judgment calls, and judgment calls are difficult to make, especially when they must be made *before* data have been gathered. Nevertheless, managers in nursing are used to making judgment calls. They carry around, consciously and subconsciously, a collection of expectations about their department, the staff and themselves. Every time they walk through the department and observe people at work or review the budget or establish staffing schedules or conduct performance appraisals, they compare actual practice to their own set of expectations and make judgments.

Some criteria for monitors will simply put into writing the nurse manager's implicit expectations. Others will reflect the expectations of the nurse manager, staff nurse and administration. Recognizing their own and others' implicit expectations is perhaps the easiest component of criteria selection for nurse managers. It simply involves thought and discussion with others.

However, to be translated into criteria, expectations must be stated in *measurable* terms. Many nurse managers have difficulty writing expectations so they can be measured. There are, however, many existing sources that can provide help. The following sources frequently contain measures that can be used for criteria:

- Departmental policies and procedures

- Departmental job descriptions

- Hospital policies and procedures

- Policies and procedures from other departments

- QA, UR or productivity studies

- Previous evaluation studies

- Other departments, hospital committees and previous managers of the department at some time in the past may have studied the topic about which criteria are currently needed. The QA/UR coordinator, chairperson of the appropriate committee or department secretary may be able to provide the criteria that were used in the study and that may be adopted in toto or adapted for the present monitoring activity.

While existing internal sources are a good starting place in the search for criteria, they should not be the only sources tapped. "People are creatures of habit!" As creatures of habit, we become accustomed to doing things in a certain way, or we accept—and expect—to encounter certain long-standing problems as part of performing a specific procedure. Internal criteria sources actually may reflect habits or problems. Therefore, it is a good idea to get a "reality check" of criteria whenever possible by consulting:

- Professional literature

  Professional literature about a specific clinical area and other general professional literature often contains benchmarks or expectations related to particular monitors. Many professional organizations publish standards of nursing practice, such as the American Nurses Association, the Nurses Association of the American College of Obstetricians and Gynecologists, American Association of Critical Care Nurses, Association of Operating Room Nurses, Emergency Department Nurses Association.

- Colleagues at other institutions or managers of other departments

  By checking criteria with others, nurse managers often gain new insights about the optimal level of performance that can be achieved.

Criteria or goals should not be limited because of the belief that things will not change. Standards should be set high, especially with regard to quality. The best way to resolve long-standing problems is to call attention to them and support requests for change with data, data and more data displayed in short, easy-to-understand reports.

Documenting The Specifications For Monitors

The Agenda of Department Monitors form on pages 120-121 provides a convenient way of recording the specifications for monitors. By recording in one place all the monitors that are being conducted in the department and the details for each monitor, the manager can document his/her entire monitoring program for administration and surveyors.

Review And Comment By The Hospital QA Committee

One of the main tasks of the hospital QA committee is to coordinate and integrate Agendas of Department Monitors hospital-wide. Without such coordination and integration, the goals of the hospital's QA program—and the JCAH QA standard—cannot be met. The QA committee consequently will evaluate each Agenda of Department Monitors to:

1. Identify similar topics

   Example

   The Agenda for the medical-surgical department in nursing in one hospital indicated that the nurse manager planned to monitor the turnaround time for STAT blood glucose and electrolyte tests. The Agenda for the laboratory had the monitoring of

Agenda of Department Monitors

TOPIC OF MONITOR	DATA TO BE COLLECTED	DATA SOURCES	FREQUENCY & AMOUNT OF DATA COLLECTION

CONTENT AND FREQUENCY OF SUMMARY REPORTS	DURATION Start/Stop/ Reappraise	PERSON TO COLLECT AND SUMMARIZE DATA	CRITERIA TO EVALUATE SUMMARY DATA & INITIATE FURTHER INVESTIGATION	CRITERIA SOURCES

turnaround times for all STAT orders as a priority item. To avoid duplication of data-gathering efforts, the hospital's QA committee suggested that the departments form a joint task force to conduct monitoring of turnaround time for all STAT orders for laboratory tests.

2. Assure that high-priority topics and responsibilities are addressed first and with appropriate frequency

Examples

In its monthly telephone survey of discharged patients, a hospital QA committee noted a pattern of concerns expressed by patients with surgical and oncological conditions. The surgical patients felt inadequately prepared to care for their wounds and left the hospital with unanswered questions about permissible activities at home. The oncological patients were confused about their schedule of medications, side effects of chemotherapy and radiation treatment and outpatient agencies who could give psychological support to them and their families. Therefore, the hospital QA committee requested that the nursing department immediately initiate a monitor on the timeliness of discharge planning done by primary nurses for patients with surgical and oncological conditions rather than beginning the monitor in three months as originally scheduled.

The nursing department of one hospital requested that the medical record department randomly select a week every six months and note the rate of incomplete admission assessments done by nurses. A number of incomplete assessments were found on the medical records during the JCAH visit. As a result the hospital QA committee requested that the nursing department increase to monthly its frequency of data collection and reports on the completion of the assessments.

3. Identify patterns of problems that should be added to an Agenda

Example

After the infection control nurse in one institution reported that the infection rates for patients who had central venous lines was increasing, the QA committee requested that nursing units who had patients on central lines begin monitoring staff adherence to procedures regarding the proper maintenance and care of the lines.

4. Identify mechanisms through which evaluation groups can provide information to one another

Example

The QA committee suggested that the nursing department share the results of its monitor on the timeliness of discharge planning for surgical and oncological patients with the social services department in the hospital. The committee felt that the monitor would uncover areas of concern that would need to be addressed by both departments to improve the effectiveness of discharge planning for these patients.

Summary

The specifications of a monitor delineate the parameters of the chosen topics so it addresses a high priority issue of the department or hospital and offers objective guidelines on which decisions can be made. Setting the specifications for the chosen topics of monitors requires the thought, ingenuity and time of nursing staff and managers. Without this careful planning "up front", energy and resources may be wasted in the collection of inaccurate or insufficient data, preparation of incomplete or untimely reports and implementation of actions based on unsubstantiated or incorrect decisions. To organize the specifications of the monitors, an Agenda of Departmental Monitors can be created using the format explained in the text chapter.

9: Completing an Agenda of Department Monitors

The specifications for selected monitors can be organized by using the Agenda of Department Monitors form found on pages 126-127. In the creation of this agenda, the nurse manager commits the department to a monitoring plan of approximately one year to promote timely reevaluation yet permit sufficient time to collect the needed data and act on identified problems. If the monitoring effort in the nursing department is primarily decentralized, each clinical unit or cluster of similar units must have an individual Agenda. All Agendas then must be submitted to a central, coordinating body, such as the QA coordinator in nursing and the nursing QA committee. This central group will provide feedback to individual units to assure that the topics with the highest priority for the entire department will be addressed without any duplication of effort. It also will coordinate the monitoring program in nursing with hospital-wide monitoring activities.

To complete an Agenda of Department Monitors, nurse managers should follow these simple steps, first at the unit and then at the departmental level:

1. **Complete the Unit/Department Monitoring Profile**

    Using the blank forms on pages 213 to 223, nurse managers should prepare a Unit/Department Monitoring Profile for each category and subcategory of monitors by recording the monitors that are currently being conducted in the department.

2. **Review the list of topics**

    Nurse managers should look at the list of potential monitoring topics for nursing in Chapters 6 and 10 and identify, for each category and subcategory, alternative/additional topics that may be appropriate for the monitoring program at the unit or departmental level. These topics should be recorded on the appropriate Unit/Department Monitoring Profile.

    At the completion of this step, nurse managers will have a complete list of topics that may be included in the unit's/department's monitoring program.

Agenda of Department Monitors

TOPIC OF MONITOR	DATA TO BE COLLECTED	DATA SOURCES	FREQUENCY & AMOUNT OF DATA COLLECTION

CONTENT AND FREQUENCY OF SUMMARY REPORTS	DURATION Start/Stop/ Reappraise	PERSON TO COLLECT AND SUMMARIZE DATA	CRITERIA TO EVALUATE SUMMARY DATA & INITIATE FURTHER INVESTIGATION	CRITERIA SOURCES

3.   Choose high-priority topics

Nurse managers, in conjunction with the nursing staff, should identify the current and potential topics that will yield the most productive information about their unit or the entire department. (See Chapter 7 for guidelines on the selection of high-priority topics.) The number of priority topics selected by each unit or cluster of units in a decentralized monitoring system should not place excessive demands on available resources, and the topics should focus on issues of specific importance to that area.

The list of priority topics generated by the units or clusters of units should be reviewed by the central coordinating group for the nursing department's monitoring program. This review ensures that the specifications for monitoring topics which have been chosen by several areas will not be developed in isolation and that topics of importance to the unit or department will not be overlooked. Once priority topics for each unit and the department have been finalized, nurse managers can proceed to Step 4.

4.   Study the sample Agenda of Department Monitors

The sample Agendas of Department Monitors on pages 130 to 159 was completed so nurse managers could get an idea of the degree of detail that is needed for each specification. The topics on the sample Agenda are representative of the topics that were suggested by nurse managers in individual interviews and by the nursing literature. Many of the topics involve issues that are complex, difficult to evaluate and have not been widely addressed in monitoring efforts in nursing. The specifications for these topics demonstrate a wide variety of approaches that can be taken to confront such issues. Rather than accept these specifications as *the* way to monitor the respective topics, nurse managers should use the information on the sample Agenda to stimulate ideas for innovative and creative ways of successfully tackling the complex issues in *their* department.

(For additional guidance on how to write specifications, see Chapter 8.)

5.   Complete an Agenda of Department Monitors for the unit/department

From the Unit/Department Monitoring Profile, nurse managers should transfer the high-priority topics that were approved by the clinical units and the central coordinating group to an Agenda of Department Monitors form and fill in each column of the Agenda to write specifications for all the topics.

To organize the monitors, nurse managers may wish to list at the top of each agenda the specific category of monitors to which the topic belongs.

6.   Share the final Agendas from the clinical units with the nursing QA committee and QA coordinator in nursing.

Once a composite Agenda has been approved by the central coordinating group in nursing, it should be given to the QA coordinator for the hospital and the hospital-wide QA committee for their input.

Closing the Loop

The completion of an Agenda of Department Monitors is a significant step toward creating the necessary nursing data base that is critical to meet the challenges and pressures in today's health care industry. However, a comprehensive system of monitors is insufficient to meet the entire scope of responsibilities related to assuring the quality of departmental services and the requirements of regulatory and accrediting agencies such as JCAH. To "close the loop", nurse managers must establish a data tracking and control management system. Such a system assists nurse managers to:

- Report, document and track data generated by monitors

- Identify problems surfaced by monitors and track the resolution of problems

- Integrate the department's quality review activities with the facility-wide program

- Display achievements of the program clearly and efficiently

- Report data systematically to the QA coordinator so it can be analyzed for patterns

- Highlight significant departmental issues

A data tracking and control management system is discussed in detail in several books published by Care Communications, Inc.,including

Solutions: Integrate, Simplify, Monitor Quality Assurance/Risk Management Activities

QA/RM: A Nurses Perspective

The Quality Assurance Status Report is recommended for use in such a system and can be found on pages 160 to 161.

Nurse managers, after reviewing the principles and organization of the data tracking and control management system in the references cited, can begin by organizing a notebook into seven sections, one for each category of monitor. Each topic on the Agenda of Department Monitors is put on a Quality Assurance Status Report and placed in the appropriate section of the notebook. Data and actions related to the monitor are then tracked until the monitor is discontinued or an identified problem is resolved. Persons responsible for followup are identified on the form so neither a monitor nor a problem is "lost" in the day-to-day departmental operations.

The notebook serves as a log which quickly demonstrates to surveyors from JCAH and other regulatory and accrediting agencies that there is a total system for departmental quality review, one that scans the services of the department, pinpoints significant patient care problems and monitors the problems through to resolution.

Agenda of Department Monitors

TOPIC OF MONITOR	DATA TO BE COLLECTED	DATA SOURCES	FREQUENCY & AMOUNT OF DATA COLLECTION
Timeliness of dis-continunance of q 4h vital signs (BP, P, R) in postoperative patients 18 years and older	For patients having general or gynecological surgery who have orders for q 4h vital signs continued beyond the first 24 hours postoperatively, identify cases in which: o Vital signs were within normal range for the patient on the final reading of initial 24 hours and o Vital signs were consistently WNL for period of continued monitoring and o No other disease process was present for which q 4h vital signs were warranted and o No postoperative complication developed Profile cases by: - Total cases reviewed - Surgeon - Type of surgery ALSO NOTE: number of cases for which order for vital signs q 4h was still present at discharge.	Medical Record	First 50 cases for each quarter as iden-tified from OR schedule

CONTENT AND FREQUENCY OF SUMMARY REPORTS	DURATION Start/Stop/ Reappraise	PERSON TO COLLECT AND SUMMARIZE DATA	CRITERIA TO EVALUATE SUMMARY DATA & INITIATE FURTHER INVESTIGATION	CRITERIA SOURCES

The Nursing QA Committee, Utilization Review Committee and the Chief of Surgery will receive the following information each quarter of the monitor:
 	
o Total number of cases reviewed
 	
  - No. and percent by surgeon
 	
  - No. and percent by type of surgery
 	
o No. and percent of cases that fail all of the criteria
 	
  - by surgeon
 	
  - by type of surgery
 	
o No. and percent of cases that fail criteria and order for vital signs was still present at discharge
 	
  - by surgeon
 	
  - by type of surgery
	First and fourth quarters of calendar year:
	
	January - March
	
	October - December
		A utilization review nurse will collect the data.
		
		A member of the Nursing QA Committee will summarize the data.
			No more than 5% of cases having an order for vital signs q 4h beyond first 24 hours will lack justification.
			
			No individual surgeon will have more than 5% of cases without justification.
			
			No cases will have orders for vital signs q 4h still present at discharge.
			
			Monitoring results that do not meet these criteria will be referred to the Chief of Surgery for review. Individual cases that fail criteria will also be referred, if requested.
				Professional judgment

Agenda of Department Monitors

TOPIC OF MONITOR	DATA TO BE COLLECTED	DATA SOURCES	FREQUENCY & AMOUNT OF DATA COLLECTION
Adequacy of nursing staff needed to execute medical and nursing orders NOTE: This monitor presupposes that nursing orders contain specified times and frequencies with which duties are to be done.	For each shift, list: o Any missed medical or nursing order for which nursing personnel were responsible o Frequency of missed orders o Any delayed medical or nursing order for which nursing personnel were responsible o Frequency of delays o Category of nursing personnel who is qualified to complete missing/delayed orders	Log maintained on each clinical unit in the study	All orders in 21 consecutive shifts

CONTENT AND FREQUENCY OF SUMMARY REPORTS	DURATION Start/Stop/ Reappraise	PERSON TO COLLECT AND SUMMARIZE DATA	CRITERIA TO EVALUATE SUMMARY DATA & INITIATE FURTHER INVESTIGATION	CRITERIA SOURCES
The nursing management committee will receive the following rpt. at the end of the monitor o Frequency and % distribution of missed/ delayed procedures/ unit and for all units by the following categories: - Basic hygiene meas. - Medication admin. - Patient/family ed - IV therapy (inc. IV meds, "regular IVs", central lines, TPN, blood trans) - Patient activity measures (eg, assistance with ambulation, ROM exercises) - Procedures related to respiratory care (C&DB, O_2, etc) - Specimen collection/ testing procedures - Psychosocial support of patient/family - Sterile procedures (eg, dressing changes, catheterizations tracheostomy care) - Assessments - Special therapies (eg, tube feedings, decubitus care, etc) - Other (specify) o Total no. of missed/ delayed procedures distributed by category of RN personnel with minimal level of credentials required to perform it.	1 week in October Repeat for one week the following March	Individual staff nurses on each unit will maintain a log. Head nurses for each unit will summarize unit information and send it to the nursing QA coordinator, who will prepare the final report.	The initial monitor is for the purpose of quantifying at the request of administration, delayed/missing procedures by nursing personnel to assess the impact of the staff reduction that occurred two months ago. The goal of the nursing department is to reduce to zero, by the end of the second quarter, the number of missed/delayed procedures that requires a registered nurse to perform them. (The head RN of each unit in study will receive a unit-specific summary to facilitate follow-up.)	Professional judgment Standards of nursing from professional organization

Agenda of Department Monitors

TOPIC OF MONITOR	DATA TO BE COLLECTED	DATA SOURCES	FREQUENCY & AMOUNT OF DATA COLLECTION
Completeness/accuracy of assessment of patients who had an orthopedic admitting diagnosis but who were placed on a unit that does not provide specialized orthopedic care	Note: o Number of records reviewed o Number of shifts reviewed for each patient up to a total of 9 shifts per patient (most recent 72 hours) o Number of shifts during which no assessment of orthopedic status was done o Number of shifts during which a partial assessment was done. Give the nature of the omission for the area or limb that was incompletely assessed as follows: - Identification of specific area assessed - Color - Temperature - Sensation - Blanching - Position - Flexion/extension of joints - Presence of orthopedic appliance - Peripheral pulses - Skin condition - Presence/absence of edema For each medical record with an omission, note: o Patient ID number o Date and shift of partial or omitted assessments	Medical records Data collection sheet	Every case until 30 cases have been reviewed

CONTENT AND FREQUENCY OF SUMMARY REPORTS	DURATION Start/Stop/ Reappraise	PERSON TO COLLECT AND SUMMARIZE DATA	CRITERIA TO EVALUATE SUMMARY DATA & INITIATE FURTHER INVESTIGATION	CRITERIA SOURCES
Monthly reports will be submitted to the nursing QA committee and the risk management committee with a final summary report issued after 30 cases have been reviewed. These reports will have the following information o Total number of medical records reviewed o Total number of shifts reviewed and average number of shifts per patient o Total number of omitted assessments Percent distribution of missing information (by topic) On a monthly basis each head nurse will receive a report of the following information from the cases that were reviewed on his/her unit o Patient ID number o Date and type of omission	Time to reach 30 cases for review Start September Repeat three months after any necessary corrective actions are taken.	Staff nurse in utilization review	The completeness of the orthopedic assessment on each shift should be 100%	Nursing standard developed by staff nurses and managers of the orthopedic unit with input from the medical staff

Agenda of Department Monitors

TOPIC OF MONITOR	DATA TO BE COLLECTED	DATA SOURCES	FREQUENCY & AMOUNT OF DATA COLLECTION

Appropriateness and attainment of goals for mobility and self care established for frail elderly who have undergone major surgery.	For cases of patients 75 years of age or older who have undergone major surgery, note the following by
	
	- Total cases reviewed
	- Total by nursing unit
	
	1. Did nursing goals relate to
	   - mobility?
	   - self-care?
	
	2. Were nursing goals met at time of discharge for
	   - mobility?
	   - self-care?
	
	3. If goals were not met:
	
	   a. Did a complication develop that interferred with goal attainment? If so, list complication.
	
	   b. Were goals set too high for patient?
	
	   c. Was follow-up care recommended?
		Medical Record
		
		Kardex
			Four cases each month from each unit caring for these patients.

CONTENT AND FREQUENCY OF SUMMARY REPORTS	DURATION Start/Stop/ Reappraise	PERSON TO COLLECT AND SUMMARIZE DATA	CRITERIA TO EVALUATE SUMMARY DATA & INITIATE FURTHER INVESTIGATION	CRITERIA SOURCES
The Nursing QA Committee and Professional Practice Committee will receive a quarterly report with the following information displayed by: o unit o No. of cases in which goals did not relate to: - mobility - self-care o No. of cases in which goals were not met at time of discharge for: - mobility - self-care o Distribution of above cases by: - No. developing complication, - by type - No. for which goal set too high - No. for whom follow-up care was recommended Each head nurse from participating units will receive a report.	One year: October 1 to September 30	One nurse per unit from PM shift will collect data during first and third quarters, night shift will collect during second and fourth quarters. Clinical nurse specialist in gerontology will summarize and analyze data and review with two members of the Professional Practice Committee before reports distributed.	100% of cases reviewed should have nursing goals related to mobility and self-care. No more than 20% of cases total and by unit should show failure to achieve goals due to inappropriate goal setting. By the end of the fourth quarter, this should be reduced to 10%. If initial goals are met in 95% or more of patients, cases will be reviewed to determine whether initial goals were set too low.	Professional Nurse Practice Committee

Agenda of Department Monitors

TOPIC OF MONITOR	DATA TO BE COLLECTED	DATA SOURCES	FREQUENCY & AMOUNT OF DATA COLLECTION

Accuracy of performance of Accucheck procedure for blood glucose by nursing personnel	Note:
	
	o Number of Accuchecks done per unit per nurse
	
	o Number of Accuchecks done in-correctly by type of discrepancy, ie, episodes of incorrect:
	
	   - Blood sample collections
	   - Preparation of strips
	   - Timing
	   - Calibration/reading of machine
	
	o Number of Accuchecks done correctly (by nurse)
	
	o Number of Accuchecks done incorrectly (by nurse)
		Log of Accucheck Procedures	All cases on one day per week picked at random

CONTENT AND FREQUENCY OF SUMMARY REPORTS	DURATION Start/Stop/ Reappraise	PERSON TO COLLECT AND SUMMARIZE DATA	CRITERIA TO EVALUATE SUMMARY DATA & INITIATE FURTHER INVESTIGATION	CRITERIA SOURCES
The following information will be submitted to the nursing QA committee monthly: o Total number of accuchecks done o Number and percent done correctly o Number and percent done incorrectly (by type of discrepancy) Each clinical unit in the monitor will receive the following information monthly. o Number of nurses who performed the procedure accurately o Number of times each nurse performed the procedure accurately o Number of nurses who did not perform the procedure accurately o Number of nurses who still must be observed	Continue until all nurses on all shifts have done 2 consecutive Accuchecks correctly. Reevaluate every 6 months after that.	Nurse educator for unit and assistant clinical nurse manager	The adherence to the procedure by nursing personnel will be 100%. Any discrepancies in performance of staff nurses on a unit will be followed up by the nurse educator for the unit.	Professional judgment of director of clinical laboratory and the nursing QA committee

Agenda of Department Monitors

TOPIC OF MONITOR	DATA TO BE COLLECTED	DATA SOURCES	FREQUENCY & AMOUNT OF DATA COLLECTION
Appropriateness and efficacy of nursing interventions for patients who have the nursing diagnosis of sleep/rest deprivation	For each patient with a current diagnosis of sleep/rest deprivation who has been receiving nursing therapy for at least 48 hours, note: o Patient ID number o Presence of the following types of nursing intervention included on the nursing care plan: - spacing of patient care to allow for rest between periods of activity - Reduction of external stimuli (eg, noise control, bright lights, excessive visitors,etc) - Provision of comfort measures (eg, backrub, position change, etc) - Provision for pain control - Stress reduction measures (eg, breathing exercises, biofeedback, etc) - Use of sedatives and/or sleep medication - Other (list specifically) For each case reviewed, scan the last 72 hours of nursing documentation, and note the number of times each day that a notation indicates the patient is sleeping or resting or that the patient states he/she is resting or sleeping better. For each case reviewed, note the patient's answers to the following questions: 1."Are you feeling more rested today than you felt during the last couple of days?" 2."Are you able to sleep better today than you were over the last couple of days?" 3."What do you feel has helped you rest or sleep better over the past several days?"	Medical records (ie, nursing care plan and nurses progress notes) Patient interviews	All cases for six months

CONTENT AND FREQUENCY OF SUMMARY REPORTS	DURATION Start/Stop/ Reappraise	PERSON TO COLLECT AND SUMMARIZE DATA	CRITERIA TO EVALUATE SUMMARY DATA & INITIATE FURTHER INVESTIGATION	CRITERIA SOURCES
The following reports will be submitted to the professional nurse practice committee monthly: o Total number of cases reviewed o Frequency and percent distribution of the types of nursing intervention o Cumulative frequency of notations of improved sleep/rest for each case o Frequency and percent distribution of patient's responses to first two interview questions o List of patient responses to the third interview question categorized by the types of nursing interventions. (Any case in which patient responses do not match the categories of nursing interventions on that patient's nursing care plan will be listed separately.) A summary of all cases will be done at the end of six months.	Six months January - June	Task force of two members of the professional nurse practice committee and the QA coordinator in nursing	There shall be documented evidence of improved sleep/rest patterns in 100% of the cases. In 100% of the interviews, patients will state improvement in sleep/rest. In 100% of the cases, the patient must credit at least one type of nursing intervention as helping to improve his/her sleep/rest. Analysis of documented types of nursing intervention will be conducted to determine possible causes of success or failure to meet these criteria.	Professional judgment

Agenda of Department Monitors

TOPIC OF MONITOR	DATA TO BE COLLECTED	DATA SOURCES	FREQUENCY & AMOUNT OF DATA COLLECTION
Accuracy of performance by staff nurses of the following specialized procedures in adult special care units: o Set up and maintenance of IABP (intraaortic balloon pump) o ICP (intracranial pressure) monitoring	For each staff nurse in each unit, observe procedures and complete a checklist on his/her performance of the procedure. Note on each checklist, any deviations from established procedure.	Checklists for the procedure	Each procedure done by each staff nurse (exclusive of orientees) until all staff have been observed.

CONTENT AND FREQUENCY OF SUMMARY REPORTS	DURATION Start/Stop/ Reappraise	PERSON TO COLLECT AND SUMMARIZE DATA	CRITERIA TO EVALUATE SUMMARY DATA & INITIATE FURTHER INVESTIGATION	CRITERIA SOURCES
The nurse director for the unit should receive a quarterly report that includes: o Total number of staff nurses in the unit o Number of staff who have been observed performing each procedure o Number of staff who correctly perform each procedure A year-to-date summary will be included, starting with the second quarter. A summary of patterns of identified deviations for any procedure will be sent to the staff education department.	Continuous At the conclusion of monitoring all staff on these skills monitoring will begin on the "maintenance of arterial lines" and "trouble shooting - pacemaker."	Peers who have been evaluated and the nurse educator for the unit will collect the data, and the head nurse will summarize the data.	Staff nurses will complete the procedures with 100% accuracy. Any staff nurse who does not achieve 100% accuracy will participate in appropriate reeducation and reevaluation before being allowed to routinely perform the procedure.	Unit policies and procedures

Agenda of Department Monitors

TOPIC OF MONITOR	DATA TO BE COLLECTED	DATA SOURCES	FREQUENCY & AMOUNT OF DATA COLLECTION
Appropriateness of nursing interventions within one hour of placing an adolescent patient in seclusion	Note: o Reason for seclusion of each patient o Clinical alternatives used by nursing personnel one hour before seclusion, including: - Verbal therapy - One-to-one therapy - Administration of prn - Isolating patient from milieu in a non-seclusion setting - Redirection of patient activity - Other treatment of choice as ordered by the treatment team (specify treatment) o Cases (by patient ID number) in which there was no evidence of the use of any of the above types of interventions within one hour of the patient's placement in seclusion o Number of cases in which patient's response to nursing intervention was not documented o Cases (by patient ID number) in which there was no evidence of behavior that can be considered dangerous to the patient or others immediately prior to seclusion	Seclusion log Medical records	All cases on psych/ medical health units for one month

CONTENT AND FREQUENCY OF SUMMARY REPORTS	DURATION Start/Stop/ Reappraise	PERSON TO COLLECT AND SUMMARIZE DATA	CRITERIA TO EVALUATE SUMMARY DATA & INITIATE FURTHER INVESTIGATION	CRITERIA SOURCES
The following summary report will be submitted to the nursing QA committee and the head nurse of the unit at the end of the month. o Total number of cases reviewed o Total number and percent distribution of unsuccessful nursing interventions attempted prior to seclusion o List of cases by patient ID number in which seclusion was used but there was no documented evidence of dangerous behavior prior to the use of seclusion	One month October	Clinical nurse specialist for psych/mental health unit and one staff nurse on the night shift	Evidence of alternative interventions used and patient's response prior to seclusion should be documented in all cases. Evidence of behavior that constitutes danger to the patient or others immediately prior to the use of seclusion should be documented in all cases. Failure to meet either of the criteria is the basis for action by the head nurse of the unit.	Institutional policy and procedure Professional literature

Agenda of Department Monitors

TOPIC OF MONITOR	DATA TO BE COLLECTED	DATA SOURCES	FREQUENCY & AMOUNT OF DATA COLLECTION
Adequacy of discharge teaching of patients who had major surgery	Note: o No. of patients readmitted to the hospital within 60 days of discharge for treatment of a complication resulting from surgery o No. of medical records reviewed o No. of medical records with a discharge summary o No. of medical records with an incomplete disch. teaching summary. Note specific incomplete areas, such as lack of instructions on: - Diet - Medication (action, admin.) - Level of activity - Followup visits with physician - Telephone number to use for additional help - Self-care techniques (eg, skin care, care of wound) o No. of "yes" responses to the following interview questions. 1. "Did you receive a copy of instructions for your care at home? 2. "Are the instructions: (a) Readable? (b) Understandable? (c) Complete?" 3. "Are you taking the medication prescribed for you?" (if applicable) 4. "Have you made an appointment for a followup visit to your physician?" (if applicable) Note the answers to the following questions: 1. "Tell me what you were able to eat for: (a) Breakfast? (b) lunch? (c) dinner?" 2. "Is that what you've been usually eating since your discharge?" 3. "How much activitiy are you involved in, for example, what was your schedule yesterday?" 4. "Was there any information you wish you had had prior to discharge?"	Admission department Medical records Telephone interview within three days of discharge date	10 cases per month selected randomly from 4N, 3N and 3S

CONTENT AND FREQUENCY OF SUMMARY REPORTS	DURATION Start/Stop/ Reappraise	PERSON TO COLLECT AND SUMMARIZE DATA	CRITERIA TO EVALUATE SUMMARY DATA & INITIATE FURTHER INVESTIGATION	CRITERIA SOURCES

The nursing QA committee will receive the following information quarterly:
 	
o Total number of re-admissions due to complications related to surgery
 	
o Total number of medical records reviewed
 	
o From the total records reviewed, a display (by percent) of the distribution of records with:
 	
  - No discharge teaching summary
  - Incomplete discharge teaching summaries (by type of omission)
 	
o Total number of patient interviews completed
 	
o Percent distribution of "yes" responses
 	
o Narrative summary for each of the last four questions
 	
The head nurse of each of the clinical units in the monitor will receive a copy of the data collection tools used for the medical record review of patients from his/her unit.
	Two months each quarter for two quarters
	
	October - March
		QA team member from unit/night shift will do medical record review.
		
		Nursing QA coordinator or disignee will do telephone interviews.
		
		Admissions department will forward read-mission rates to nursing QA coordinator monthly.
		
		The QA coordinator for nursing will complete the quarterly reports.
			Any patient readmitted for treatment of a complication after major surgery will be reviewed by an ad hoc committee of the nursing QA committee. If the readmission is related to the lack of appropriate discharge teaching by nursing personnel, the head nurse of the unit on which patient was originally cared for will be notified. The ad hoc committee will report any identified patterns to the staff education department for followup.
			
			Discharge teaching summaries will be completed in 100% of the cases. Failure to meet this goal will result in followup by the head nurse of the unit involved.
			
			Patients will express satisfaction with their discharge teaching summary in at least 98% of the cases. Any pattern of negative responses or comments will be referred to the professional nurse practice committee for review.
			
			Patient comments on their post-discharge care will demonstrate compliance to the prescribed regimen in 98% of the cases. If a lower rate is achieved, the matter will be investigated by the joint practice committee.
				Professional judgment of nursing QA committee and professional nurse practice committee.

Agenda of Department Monitors

TOPIC OF MONITOR	DATA TO BE COLLECTED	DATA SOURCES	FREQUENCY & AMOUNT OF DATA COLLECTION

Ability of newly diagnosed insulin-dependent diabetic patient/family member to perform select skills needed to "survive" post discharge	NOTE:
	
	o Number of cases reviewed
	o For each patient/family member in sample note:
	
	  - Deviations from mandatory steps in procedure for:
	
	    - administration of insulin
	    - home blood glucose monitoring
	
	  - Deviation from appropriate menu selection for at least one day
	
	  - Inability to state three major symptoms of hypoglycemia and hyperglycemia
	
	  - Failure to state correct treatment for hypoglycemia and hyperglycemia
	
	  - Failure to specify who to contact/what to do in an emergency
	
	For patients/family members who were unable to demonstrate competency in all skills 24 hours prior to scheduled discharge note number:
	
	  - whose attending physician was notified
	
	  - who were discharged on schedule with no evidence of plan for follow-up supervision/instruction
	
	  - whose discharge was delayed
		Observation of patient
		
		Patient interview
		
		Procedures for administration of insulin, blood glucose monitoring
		
		Education protocols for menu selection and recognition and treatment of hypoglycemia and hyperglycemia
			Review each case of newly diagnosed insulin dependent diabetics until 20 cases have been reviewed.
			
			The observations and patient interview will be done on the day preceding or the day of discharge.

CONTENT AND FREQUENCY OF SUMMARY REPORTS	DURATION Start/Stop/ Reappraise	PERSON TO COLLECT AND SUMMARIZE DATA	CRITERIA TO EVALUATE SUMMARY DATA & INITIATE FURTHER INVESTIGATION	CRITERIA SOURCES
The multidisciplinary Diabetes Advisory Task Force will receive a report after 10 cases are reviewed and again after 20 cases are reviewed. The report will include: o Total number of cases reviewed o Total number and percent of deviations distributed by skill (i.e., insulin administration, blood glucose monitoring, diet selection, treatment of hypoglycemia and hyperglycemia, and what to do in an emergency). The primary nurse for the patient will be notified of deviations at the time data is collected. o Distribution of deviations for each skill by type of deviation. o The number and percent of cases failing criteria for which physician was not notified. o The number and percent of cases failing criteria that were discharged with no evidence of plan for follow-up supervision/ instruction. o Number and percent of delayed discharges	Six months: October - March	A nurse and dietician who are members of the Diabetes Task Force.	Patients/family members will have 100% compliance for each of the following: - administration of insulin - home blood glucose monitoring - menu selection for one day - symptoms and treatment for hypoglycemia and hyperglycemia - what to do in an emergency All cases failing to comply should have evidence that the attending physician was notified, and that the patient was not discharged.	Professional literature and expert judgment

Agenda of Department Monitors

TOPIC OF MONITOR	DATA TO BE COLLECTED	DATA SOURCES	FREQUENCY & AMOUNT OF DATA COLLECTION
Outcomes of patients with nursing diagnosis of alteration in skin integrity: pressure ulcer	NOTE: o Number of cases reviewed o Presence/absence of measurable goals on nursing care plan related to this nursing diagnosis o Presence/absence of daily documentation of the following related to pressure ulcer: - location - stage - width, depth, dimension and coloration - condition of surrounding skin - presence/absence of drainage - description of drainage, if any - treatment o Presence/absence of documentation of nutritional assessment of patient o Presence/absence of documentation of daily nutritional intake of patient o Presence/absence of nutritional consultation if patient intake is inadequate to promote healing o Presence/absence of stable or decreasing size of pressure ulcer validated by observation of patient or documentation o Initiation of alternative treatment if size of pressure ulcer is not stable or decreasing within three - seven days of treatment, depending on treatment modality. o Were goals met?	Observation of patient Medical Record	All cases of patients with pressure ulcers

CONTENT AND FREQUENCY OF SUMMARY REPORTS	DURATION Start/Stop/ Reappraise	PERSON TO COLLECT AND SUMMARIZE DATA	CRITERIA TO EVALUATE SUMMARY DATA & INITIATE FURTHER INVESTIGATION	CRITERIA SOURCES
The Hospital and Nursing QA Committees will receive the following report quarterly: o Total number of cases reviewed o Total number and percent of cases having measurable goals related to the nursing diagnosis o Total number and percent of cases in which goals were met o Total number and percent of cases in which either size of pressure sore remained stable or diminished within 3 to 7 days of instituting treatment, or change in treatment was initiated o Total number and percent of cases in which a nutritional assessment was done o Total number and percent of cases in which dietary requirements were met by patient or alteration in diet plan occurred Head nurses will receive data collection sheets for patients on their units included in the sample. The supervisor of clinical dieticians will receive a summary of data related to nutritional assessment and treatment.	Two quarters per year January – March July – September	Certified enterostomal therapist/skin specialist, clinical dietician and staff nurse from Nursing QA Committee will collect and summarize data.	In 100% of the cases the size of the pressure sore should be stable or smaller within 3 to 7 days depending on treatment modality <u>or</u> initiation of new treatment is started. The goals stated in the nursing care plan that relate to the nursing diagnosis of alteration in skin integrity should be met in at least 80% of the cases. The documentation of the progress of the pressure sore is complete in at least 80% of the cases. The nutritional status of the patient is assessed and evaluated throughout treatment of the pressure sore in 90% of the cases.	Expert opinion Nursing standards for care of patients with alteration in skin integrity Dietician

Agenda of Department Monitors

TOPIC OF MONITOR	DATA TO BE COLLECTED	DATA SOURCES	FREQUENCY & AMOUNT OF DATA COLLECTION

Completeness/timeliness of documentation of IV therapy by nursing personnel	Note:
	
	o Number of IV solutions dispensed per unit
	
	o Number of charts reviewed
	
	o Number of deviations from the procedure for documenting IVs by type of deviation, including omission, inaccurate or incomplete notation concerning:
	
	  - Condition of IV site
	  - Solution infusing
	  - Rate of infusion
	  - Site change
	  - Dressing change over IV site
	  - Tubing change
	
	o Number of IV charges submitted by nursing personnel for IV solutions
		Medical records
		
		Pharmacy log
			10 cases per month per unit

CONTENT AND FREQUENCY OF SUMMARY REPORTS	DURATION Start/Stop/ Reappraise	PERSON TO COLLECT AND SUMMARIZE DATA	CRITERIA TO EVALUATE SUMMARY DATA & INITIATE FURTHER INVESTIGATION	CRITERIA SOURCES
The following information will be submitted to the nursing QA committee monthly. o Total number of medical records reviewed o Total number of IVs dispensed to the units in the monitor for one month o Total number of IV charges submitted by the units in the monitor for one month o Frequency and percent distribution of deviations (by type of deviation) A summary of the monthly reports will be done quarterly. Each clinical unit will receive a report at the time of data collection which includes: o Patient ID number for any medical record with a discrepancy o Type of discrepancy	Two quarters per year April - June October - December	Pharmacy supervisor and QA team member from each unit	The documentation of IV therapy should be: o 100% for solution, rate of infusion and condition of site o 85% for site change and dressing change o 75% for tubing change Deviations noted on a unit will be followed up by the head nurse. The number of IVs charged by the pharmacy should be the same as the number dispensed. A difference of more than 50% will be investigated further by the nursing pharmacy committee.	Departmental policies and procedures

Agenda of Department Monitors

TOPIC OF MONITOR	DATA TO BE COLLECTED	DATA SOURCES	FREQUENCY & AMOUNT OF DATA COLLECTION
Satisfaction with nurses' response to requests for pain relief by post-surgical patients and oncology patients	Note: Number of "yes" answers to the following questions and summary of any comments: 1. "Did a nurse respond to your call when you were in pain within a time period that was acceptable to you?" 2. "Did a nurse bring you pain medication if you asked for it within a time period that was acceptable to you?" 3. "Did the pain medication work as quickly as you thought it should? 4. "Did the nurse do anything else besides give you pain medication in order to make you more comfortable, such as give you a backrub or change your position?" a. "If yes, what?" b. "Did the other pain relief measure work?" 5. "Did the nurse check back with you within a half-hour to see if the pain medication or other measures had worked?" 6. "Was there anything you wished had been done to control pain, but wasn't?" 7. "Do you have any further comments or suggestions regarding your pain control by nursing personnel?"	Patient Interviews	Interview on their second post-operative day all patients who had major surgery and a 10% sample of oncology patients. Do this one day per week until 25 cases for each patient group have been obtained.

CONTENT AND FREQUENCY OF SUMMARY REPORTS	DURATION Start/Stop/ Reappraise	PERSON TO COLLECT AND SUMMARIZE DATA	CRITERIA TO EVALUATE SUMMARY DATA & INITIATE FURTHER INVESTIGATION	CRITERIA SOURCES

The following information will be submitted to the nursing QA committee on a monthly basis until all interviews are complete.
 	
o Number of interviews completed for sugical patients and for oncology patients
 	
For the total sample and for each type of patient sample:
 	
o Percent of "yes" responses to each question
 	
o Overall percent of "yes" responses to interview questions
 	
o Summary of comments divided into three areas:
 	
  - Informational comments
  - Positive comments
  - Critical comments
	One quarter
	
	October - December
	
	Repeat after any plan of action is instituted to address an identified problem
		Representative from pastoral care and one of the nurses from staff and patient education will collect the data.
		
		An ad hoc committee of the nursing QA committee will summarize the results, recommend follow-up actions and conduct subsequent monitorings if necessary.
			The rate of "yes" responses to each question for each patient group should be at least 95%, and the overall "yes" response rate should be 99% by end of the quarter.	Professional judgment of nursing QA committee

Agenda of Department Monitors

TOPIC OF MONITOR	DATA TO BE COLLECTED	DATA SOURCES	FREQUENCY & AMOUNT OF DATA COLLECTION
Efficacy of a "falls reduction program" in nursing services	Note number of falls reported by: o Unit o Age of patient o Shift o Type of injury (ie, no injury, minor injury, major injury/ fracture) o Place of fall o Activity of the patient at the time of the fall (ie, walking, lying in bed, sitting in chair) o Condition of patient (ie, alert and oriented, confused/disoriented, semi- or unconscious, sedated) Note preventive measures used by nursing personnel present at the time of the fall (by type of measure): o Siderails up o Restraints on o Medication given to induce sedation o Frequent observation	Incident reports Medical records Interviews of nurses assigned to patients	All cases of patient falls reported daily on all shifts.

CONTENT AND FREQUENCY OF SUMMARY REPORTS	DURATION Start/Stop/ Reappraise	PERSON TO COLLECT AND SUMMARIZE DATA	CRITERIA TO EVALUATE SUMMARY DATA & INITIATE FURTHER INVESTIGATION	CRITERIA SOURCES
The following information will be sent to the nursing QA committee and safety committee monthly, with an overall summary at the end of the quarter. o Total number of falls reported o Percent distribution of falls according to each variable on which data were collected o Percent distribution documented preventive measures at the time of the fall (by type of measure) At the end of the quarter, a copy of the final report will be sent to the head nurses of the units cited in the report.	Three quarters October-June	Risk manager and "house" supervisor on whose shift the fall occurs will collect data. The risk manager will prepare summary reports.	A reduction of 50% in the rate of reported falls, as compared to the rate prior to the "falls reduction program." Failure to meet this goal will result in a reevaluation of the "falls reduction program."	Professional judgment of the risk manager and nursing QA committee Professional literature

Agenda of Department Monitors

TOPIC OF MONITOR	DATA TO BE COLLECTED	DATA SOURCES	FREQUENCY & AMOUNT OF DATA COLLECTION

Outcomes of patients on clinical units who receive cardiopulmonary resuscitation.	Note each item by:
	
	- total receiving CPR
	- number of inpatients
	- number in emergency room only
	
	1. Resuscitations in which patient was:
	
	  - resuscitated
	  - alive 6 hours past CPR
	  - discharged alive
	
	2. Number of patients alive 6 hours past CPR and there was:
	
	  - no apparent change in neurological status
	  - change in neurological status apparently related to CPR
	  - unknown
	
	3. Number of patients subsequently discharged alive and at discharge there was :
	
	  - no apparent change in neurological status
	  - change in neurological status apparently related to CPR
	  - unknown
		Medical Record	All reported resuscitations

	For patients who exhibited change in neurological status or who expired, note whether there were deviations from CPR protocol recorded on CPR report sheet.	CPR report sheet	

CONTENT AND FREQUENCY OF SUMMARY REPORTS	DURATION Start/Stop/ Reappraise	PERSON TO COLLECT AND SUMMARIZE DATA	CRITERIA TO EVALUATE SUMMARY DATA & INITIATE FURTHER INVESTIGATION	CRITERIA SOURCES
The multidisciplinary CPR Committee should receive quarterly report that displays: o Total number and percent of CPRs o Total number and percent - inpatient - emergency room for the information requested in Data to be Collected. Report should show current quarter's statistics and compare with most recent four quarters. Report should also be sent to Director of Nursing, Nursing QA Committee and Hospital QA Committee.	Continuous	Nurse from QA department serving on CPR Committee	At least 40% of patients should be alive 6 hours post CPR. At least 20% of patients should be discharged alive. CPR Committee will review all cases in which: - patient was resuscitated but expired within 6 hours - patient was alive 6 hrs post CPR, and expired prior to discharge - neurological deficit was present at any time and the CPR protocol was not followed.	Professional literature and baseline established for hospital after review of one year's statistics

Quality Assurance

TYPE OF PROBLEM

DATE & SOURCE	SPECIFIC PROBLEM,	CAUSE AND ATTRIBUTION	ACTION		RESP. PARTY
			WHAT	WHEN	

Status Report

NEXT REVIEW DATE	STATUS AND FURTHER ACTION	NEXT REVIEW DATE	STATUS AND FURTHER ACTION	NEXT REVIEW DATE	STATUS AND FURTHER ACTION	DATE SOLVED

10: Topics For Monitors For Specific Clinical Areas

The monitoring topics listed in Chapter 6 can be used in any clinical area in the hospital. Most of the topics are relevant for general medical/surgical areas, and many of them are also appropriate for specialized clinical units. However, clusters of clinical areas must have topics specifically tailored for them. These topics must be included in the Agenda of Department Monitors for the unit as well as the master Agenda of Department Monitors for the nursing department to meet the regulatory requirements of JCAH and to amass the kind of data base that is necessary for effective unit/departmental management.

Through interviews with nurse managers, clinical nurse specialists and staff nurses from specialized clinical areas and a review of the professional literature related to these areas, lists of monitoring topics for five special clinical areas have been developed:

1. Maternal/child health
    Part A: maternal/newborn   pp 164 to 173
    Part B: pediatrics   pp 174 to 177

2. Special care   pp 178 to 183

3. Psychiatry-mental health   pp 184 to 190

4. Operating room/recovery room   pp 191 to 198

5. Emergency department   pp 199 to 205

The specialized areas have been classified according to a "medical model," since an accepted "nursing model" has not yet evolved nationally. However, the classifications can be rearranged to fit the organization of clinical units within a particular hospital.

Topics in the five special clinical areas have been grouped under the seven major categories of monitors described in this book. The topics are not intended to be viewed as an exhaustive compendium of all possible subjects for monitoring in the specialized areas. However, they can serve as guides for choosing topics that are relevant to a specific unit and they can be used in planning a comprehensive monitoring program at both the unit and departmental levels.

Maternal/Newborn

Category I.   Utilization Monitors

Subcategory A.   Statistical Distribution Related to Orders, Referrals and Costs

- Distribution of normal and at-risk patients admitted per day/week/month

- Distribution of at-risk patients who were identified after admission

- Distribution of mothers/infants admitted to the inpatient unit from an outpatient obstetrical area (by physician)

- Distribution of patients' utilization of services/facilities, including:

    -prenatal instruction
    -birthing/labor and delivery rooms
    -specific inpatient care area (eg, antepartum, nursery, postpartum, etc)
    -outpatient obstetrical services
    -short-stay areas

- Distribution of specialized diagnostic procedures (eg, non-stress tests (NTS), oxytocin challenge test (OCT), ultrasound, etc)

- Distribution of surgical procedures performed in the labor and delivery area by:

    -type of surgery (eg, episiotomy, repair of episiotomy, type of laceration repaired)
    -physician
    -shift/day/week/month

- Distribution of deliveries by type, including:

    -forceps (eg, high, medium and low outlet)
    -spontaneous vaginal (include delivery position)
    -C-section

- Distribution of indications for C-section

- Distribution of types of analgesia/anesthesia used during labor

- Distribution of types of anesthesia used during delivery

- Average length of stay of patients in the recovery area after delivery

- Average length of stay of infants with mothers after delivery

- Distribution of non-routine neonatal procedures (by type)

Category I.   Utilization Monitors

Subcategory B.   Clinical Appropriateness and Timeliness of Admissions, Orders and Referrals

- Physicians' compliance to criteria for admitting mothers to and using birthing rooms

- Physicians' compliance to criteria for discharging/transferring mothers from the recovery room (by physician)

Category I.   Utilization Monitors

Subcategory C.   Clinicians' Use of Assessments and Recommendations Made by Staff Nurses, Clinical Nurse Specialists or Nurse Managers

- Appropriate and timely use of nurses' preadmission assessment of the following:

  -educational needs and/or preparation of the pregnant woman and her family
  -maternal/infant risk status
  -parental desires and priorities regarding the manner in which labor and birth
   should be conducted
  -parents' coping skills

Category II.   Departmental Performance Monitors

Subcategory A.   Overall Departmental Performance Monitors

- Average hours of nursing care per patient per shift in:

  -labor and delivery
  -newborn area
  -postpartum area

Category II.   Departmental Performance Monitors

Subcategory B.   Performance of Specific Departmental Functions Involving Direct Patient Care

- Timeliness of notification of physicians of patients' admissions by nursing personnel

- Accuracy and completeness of the nursing assessments of the mothers-to-be immediately after admission or during the antepartal period, including:

  -reason for admission
  -patient and family understanding of the admitting diagnosis
  -previous pregnancies and outcomes
  -gestational age of fetus
  -prenatal course

- Accuracy and completeness of the nursing assessment of the fetus at the time of admission of the mother-to-be and during the antepartal period, including:

  -fetal heart rate (FHR)
  -fetal position and presentation

- Accuracy and completeness of ongoing assessment of the mother-to-be and fetus by nurses throughout the antepartal period

- Timeliness of assessments of the patients' status throughout the labor/delivery process, including:

  -uterine contractions
  -FHR
  -tolerance of labor
  -progress of labor

- Competence of staff nurses in providing support to the patients' primary support person(s) during labor

- Accuracy and timeliness of evaluation by nursing personnel of changes in the patients' risk status during labor

- Completeness of the nursing assessments of the intrapartal patients, including:

  -basic education and understanding of instruction given during prenatal classes
  -socio-cultural considerations
  -patient expectations and goals of childbirth
  -vital signs and review of body systems
  -history of recent infection
  -time and type of last meal
  -present emotional status
  -presence/absence of support person(s)
  -fetal size, position and presentation, dilation and effacement of cervix, station
   of presenting part
  -FHR
  -onset, frequency and duration of contractions
  -presence/absence of ruptured membranes
  -presence/absence of vaginal bleeding or discharge

- Competence of nursing personnel in the management of abnormal occurrences during the intrapartal period, including:

  -hypertensive crisis
  -tetanic contractions
  -fetal distress
  -fetal demise
  -precipitous delivery
  -maternal death
  -emergency C-section

-multiple births
-utero-placental insufficiency
-prolapsed cord
-maternal thromboemboli
-hemorrhage

- Appropriateness, timeliness and completeness of assessments of the post-partum patients by nurses, including:

-condition of breast, nipple
-condition of perineum
-location/condition of fundus
-amount and description of lochia
-bowel and bladder function
-circulatory status
-vital signs
-nutritional/fluid status
-bonding between mother and infant, family interactional patterns, adjustment
 of mother to new role

- Accuracy and timeliness of nurses' management of adverse occurrences in postpartum patients, including:

-hemorrhage
-shock
-coma
-neurological emergencies
-emboli

- Timeliness, appropriateness and completeness of initial assessment of the newborn, including:

-airway patency
-APGAR scoring
-physical status, especially presence of any anomalies
-neurological status and reactivity
-gestational age
-need for temperature maintenance
-behavioral state

- Timeliness, appropriateness and completeness of nursing assessment of infants during the hospital stay, including:

-physical status, especially presence of any anomalies
-behavioral characteristics and interactional capabilities
-developmental characteristics
-parental care
-nutritional status
-feeding patterns

-any adverse effects from drugs
-vital signs, weight, review of body systems
-uterine tone and presence/absence of contractions
-uterine size, fundal height
-presence/absence of ruptured membranes
-elimination patterns
-pattern of weight loss/gain
-presence/absence of jaundice

- Staff nurses' adherence to policies regarding thermoregulation of the newborn with priority placed on maternal-infant contact as the method of thermoregulation

- Accuracy and timeliness of staff nurses' performance of specialized skills in the nursery, such as:

    -infant physical examination
    -bulb and DeLee suctioning
    -infant resuscitation
    -nasogastric lavage/gavage
    -eye care
    -cord care
    -developmental assessment
    -infant feeding
    -use of incubators and other thermoregulatory equipment
    -use of phototherapy equipment
    -use of cardiorespiratory monitors
    -management of parenteral therapy

- Accuracy, completeness and timeliness of staff nurses' performance of specialized procedures, including:

    -abdominal examination for fetal size, position and station
    -monitoring of uterine contractions via palpation
    -administration of tocolytic and oxytocic drugs
    -monitoring of FHR by auscultation
    -positioning the mother for labor and birth
    -vaginal exams
    -application and placement of tocodynamometer
    -application of fetal scalp electrodes
    -application and placement of external HR detector
    -interpretation of fetal monitor strips
    -maintenance of patency of infant's airway
    -resuscitation of the newborn
    -eye/cord care of newborn
    -proper identification of newborn
    -initiation of bonding between infant and parent
    -palpation of uterine fundus

    -inspection/evaluation of lochia

- Accuracy, completeness and timeliness of implementation of appropriate nursing care protocols for specific high and low-risk maternal/infant situations (eg, postpartum hemorrhage, neonatal hypoglycemia, normal labor, OCT, NST, CST, etc)

- Accuracy, completeness and timeliness of implementation of nursing care protocols for specific high and low-risk infant situations (eg, triage/admission care, cardiorespiratory emergencies, thermal and metabolic problems, jaundice, etc)

- Appropriateness and timeliness of staff nurses' management of mothers whose babies were stillborn or who have died

- Appropriateness and timeliness of staff nurses' management of babies with congenital defects

- Appropriateness and timeliness of staff nurses' management of mothers with babies who have congenital defects

- Appropriateness and timeliness of staff nurses' management of mothers experiencing difficulty with infant acquaintance, attachment and bonding

- Completeness and timeliness of communication between maternal and infant caregivers concerning:

    -number and type of anticipated deliveries
    -number and nature of high-risk patients
    -mutual needs of mothers and infants

- Completeness of patients' knowledge of the following after instruction by nursing personnel:

    -parent/child attachment
    -infant care
    -breast feeding
    -bottle feeding
    -breast care
    -mother's selfcare during involution process

- Accuracy and completeness of staff nurses' knowledge of:

    -maternal and newborn physiology and pathophysiology
    -alternative childbirth practices and settings
    -family-centered care
    -parent-infant relationships
    -newborn behavior
    -application of fetal monitoring equipment
    -interpretation of fetal heart rate patterns
    -appropriate interventions in obstetrical/newborn emergencies
    -assistance with cesarean birth

-use and application of ultrasonography

- Accuracy and completeness of staff knowledge of calculating and preparing drugs for administration to infants

Category II.   Departmental Performance Monitors

Subcategory C.   Availability, Distribution and Appropriateness of Use of Departmental Resources

- Availability of staff to provide coverage on above-average census days and/or during variable census periods within shifts

- Appropriateness of nursing staff schedule/assignment based on risk criteria used to assess patients' care needs

- Availability of drugs needed for maternal/infant care

- Availability of sterile supplies for deliveries

- Availability of equipment and supplies to provide infant care

- Presence/functional integrity of equipment for:

  -gynecologic exams
  -amniocentesis
  -maternal/fetal monitoring
  -ultrasonography

- Adequacy/functional integrity of nursery equipment for:

  -neonatal CPR
  -phototherapy
  -intubation
  -incubation
  -isolation of infected infants
  -infant transfer

Category II.   Departmental Performance Monitors

Subcategory D. Documentation

- Completeness and timeliness of documentation of nursing diagnosis for normal and at-risk mothers, infants and families

- Completeness of documentation by nursing personnel of:

  -parents' emotional status
  -family dynamics
  -parents' knowledge of the care and handling of the newborn
  -parenting skills and infant stimulation
  -nutrition

- Timeliness of documentation of the collection and disposition of neonates' specimens (urine, blood, etc)

- Timeliness and completeness of documentation on special flow sheets used in maternal/infant care

Category III.   User Satisfaction Monitors

- Mother's satisfaction with nursing assistance during labor/birth

- Mother's satisfaction with rooming-in facilities and process

- Mother's satisfaction with nursing assistance for herself and her infant throughout the hospital stay

- Mother's satisfaction with instruction on the care and handling of the newborn

- Mother's satisfaction with the amount and availability of contact with her infant

- Mother's satisfaction with instruction on self-care, particularly regarding breast feeding and the management of lactation

- Family's/support person's satisfaction with nursing care and institutional policies regarding the care of the mother and infant

- Physicians' satisfaction with the nursing care of obstetrical patients and their families

Category IV.   Safety Monitors

- Accuracy of mother/infant identification by nursing personnel

- Staff's compliance with handwashing and/or gowning procedures prior to contact with mothers and/or infants

- Appropriateness and timeliness of reporting of suspected infection in mothers and/or infants

- Staff's adherence to maternal/infant isolation procedures

- Appropriateness and timeliness of cleaning of cribs between infants

- Appropriateness and timeliness of cleaning of labor and delivery areas and equipment between mothers

Category V.   Quality Control Monitors

- Timeliness, thoroughness of equipment checks for electrical hazards in maternal/infant care area

Category VI.   Incident/Occurrence Monitors

- Deliveries that were unattended by a physician with OB privileges

- Maternal/infant deaths

- Hospital-acquired maternal/neonatal infections

- Maternal/fetal complications that followed administration of anesthesia during the first or second stage of labor

- Fetal distress identified during the first or second stage of labor

- Infants with APGAR scores below 6 at one minute and/or below 8 at five minutes

- Fetal injury during birth (by type, eg: skull fracture, paralysis, brachial palsy, etc)

- Newborns admitted or transferred to a newborn ICU for complications that developed during birth

- Newborns transferred to a neonatal ICU for complications that occurred during the immediate neonatal period

- Newborn resuscitation attempts and their success rate

- Neonatal jaundice that requires phototherapy

- Neonatal hypoglycemia or hypocalcemia requiring parenteral therapy

- Meconium aspiration

- Multiple collections of blood specimens from infants that result in skin trauma or volume depletion

- Women in the second stage of labor for more than four hours when there were no maternal/fetal complications

- Women in the third stage of labor for more than two hours with or without a retained placenta

- Prolapsed cord

- Placenta abruptio, placenta previa

- Maternal blood loss during or after labor/delivery that required a transfusion or resulted in drop in Hgb of 2.5 mg% or more

- Maternal injury or complications that occurred as a result of labor/delivery (eg, third-degree laceration, retained placenta, infection, etc)

- Length of stay of mother in the recovery room exceeding two hours and/or transfer of the mother to the ICU for complications during labor and delivery

- Unplanned return of the mother to the delivery room or surgery

- Maternal seizures or other CNS emergencies

- Maternal cardiovascular emergencies requiring resuscitation

- Inconsistency of explanation to mothers concerning infant care by the physician and the nursing staff

- Staff nurses' performance of procedures during labor and delivery that are outside the scope of nursing practice, such as:

  -rupture of membranes
  -insertion of catheters during a cutdown
  -initiation or continuation of anesthesia
  -performance of amniocentesis
  -performance of episiotomy in non-emergency situations
  -insertion of intrauterine catheters
  -performance of fetal scalp sampling

- Staff nurses' performance of procedures in the nursery that are outside their scope of practice, such as:

  -endotracheal intubation
  -initiation of peripheral and central intravascular catheters
  -administration of intravascular or intracardiac medications

- Staff nurses' performance of procedures in the postpartum area that are outside their scope of practice, such as removal of uterine packing

Category VII.   Monitors of Patient Management and Clinical Practices of Other Departments

N/A

Pediatrics

Category I.   Utilization Monitors

Subcategory A.   Statistical Distribution Related to Orders, Referrals and Costs

- Distribution of patients by age, average level of acuity, diagnosis, payor status

Category I.   Utilization Monitors

Subcategory B.   Medical Appropriateness and Timeliness of Admissions, Orders and Referrals

- Timeliness of physicians' orders after admissions of patient

- Timeliness of physicians' response to notification of a change in child's health status

Category I.   Utilization Monitors

Subcategory C.   Clinicians' Use of Assessments and Recommendations Made by Staff Nurses, Clinical Nurse Specialists or Nurse Managers

N/A

Category II.   Departmental Performance Monitors

Subcategory A.   Overall Departmental Performance Monitors

N/A

Category II.   Departmental Performance Monitors

Subcategory B.   Performance of Specific Departmental Functions Involving Direct Patient Care

- Completeness of nursing assessment of pediatric patients on admission, including:

  -history of illnesses, past hospitalizations
  -level of growth and development
  -measurement of head and chest of children under two years of age
  -parent/child patterns of interaction
  -parent/child reactions to the hospital environment
  -level of activity
  -physical assessment (eg, vital signs, height, weight, evaluation of body systems, etc)
  -level of comfort

-patterns of rest, sleep and play
-patterns of nutrition

- Completeness and accuracy of neurological assessment of children with neurological conditions

- Assessment by nursing personnel of the adequacy of nutritional intake by pediatric patients given an adult-oriented menu

- Timeliness of notification of the physician of changes in patient status that must be addressed

- Accuracy of vital signs evaluation (especially temperature and blood pressure) by staff nurses

- Appropriateness of feeding technique used by nursing personnel for infants with a cleft palate

- Staff nurses' ability to insert an IV into a scalp vein

- Staff nurses' performance of procedures for properly maintaining and caring for IV infusions in infants and children

- Accuracy of staff nurses' calculations of medication doses for infants and children

- Staff nurses' ability to perform CPR on infants/children

- Appropriateness and timeliness of nurses' referrals to agencies in the community, such as:

  -child protective services
  -family services
  -child guidance
  -public/community health

- Timeliness of nurses' referral of parents of children with chronic or debilitating conditions to designated support groups

- Timeliness and appropriateness of discharge teaching for parents (significant others) with children who have a specific type of condition, such as:

  -orthopedic problem
  -cleft palate
  -cystic fibrosis
  -rheumatic fever
  -diabetes
  -cancer
  -gastroenteritis

- Accuracy of staff nurses' performance of special procedures, including

  -preparation and maintenance of isolette
  -phototherapy
  -apnea monitoring
  -infant height and weight

- Appropriateness of nurses' play therapy program for children in different age groups (eg, preschool, elementary school age, pre-teen, etc)

- Effectiveness of nursing interventions to obtain pain control in children

Category II.   Departmental Performance Monitors

Subcategory B.   Availability, Distribution and Appropriateness of Use of Departmental Resources

- Availability of comfortable and private facilities for parents to stay overnight

- Availability of special teaching aids needed for child/family education

- Availability of equipment and supplies specialized for the pediatric patient (eg, sphygmomanometers, tourniquets, arm boards, etc)

- Maintenance of trays of properly functioning equipment for physical exams (eg, otoscopes, ophthalmascopes, reflex hammer, etc)

Category II.   Departmental Performance Monitors

Subcategory D.   Documentation

N/A

Category III.   User Satisfaction Monitors

- Parents' satisfaction with the nursing care of their children

- Parents' satisfaction with their ability to care for their child after discharge following instruction by nursing personnel

Category IV.   Safety Monitors

- Adherence of nursing personnel to safety guidelines regarding the care of infants and children, including:

  -the presence of rails and "bubbles" on cribs
  -the use of restraints while patients are in wagons, wheelchairs and high chairs
  -intensity of supervision of toddlers when patients are out of bed

- Maintenance of cleanliness and safety of toys provided on the unit for play therapy

Category V.   Quality Control Monitors

- Verification of institutional certification of nursing staff who administer chemo-therapy to children

- Timeliness and thoroughness of alarms checks on all monitoring equipment

- Maintenance of regular checks of scales

Category VI.   Incident/Occurrence Monitors

N/A

Category VIII.   Monitors of Patient Management and Clinical Practices of Other Departments

- Adequacy of supervision of pediatric patients by transport or x-ray personnel while patients are off the unit for testing

- Appropriateness and timeliness of interventions by the social worker, psycho—logist, child life specialist and/or school teacher to meet the psychosocial needs of patients/families

Special Care

Category I.   Utilization Monitors

Subcategory A.   Statistical Distribution Related to Orders, Referrals and Costs

- Distribution of patients placed in special care units by:

  -physician
  -acuity level
  -special procedures/treatments required
  -DRG
  -length of stay
  -principal diagnosis
  -number and type of secondary diagnoses

- Distribution of patients who have one-day stays in a special care unit by:

  -physician
  -DRG/diagnosis
  -number of admission criteria met
  -type of admission criteria met

- Distribution of mortality by:

  -physician
  -diagnosis/DRG
  -acuity level

- Rate of readmission to special care units

Category I.   Utilization Monitors

***Subcategory B.   Clinical Appropriateness and Timeliness of Admissions, Orders and
                    Referrals***

- Timeliness of transfer of direct-admit patients from admitting to the special care
  unit

- Appropriateness and timeliness of referrals to the clinical nurse specialist who is
  responsible for planning patient care

- Physicians' adherence to criteria for admitting patients to special care units

- Timeliness of physicians' visits to patients following admission to special care
  units

- Timeliness of physicians' response to notification of change in patients' status

- Appropriateness of physicians' orders for a Swan-Ganz catheter for patients who
  stayed in the unit only one day

- Appropriateness of physicians' orders for nurses to perform procedures for which there are no existing policies or procedures (eg, use of lidocaine wheels during intracatheter insertions, injection of morphine sulphate through an epidural catheter)

- Timeliness and appropriateness of orders for blood gases

- Physicians' adherence to criteria for discharging patients from special care units

- Timeliness of discharge of patients from special care units

- Timeliness and appropriateness of referrals of cardiac surgery patients to cardiac rehabilitation activities

Category I.   Utilization Monitors

Subcategory C.   Clinicians' Use of Nursing Assessments and Recommendations Made by Staff Nurses, Clinical Nurse Specialists or Nurse Managers

- Families' (significant others') adherence to nurses' recommendations to participate in a nurse-sponsored spouse support group in a special care unit

Category II.   Departmental Performance Monitors

Subcategory A.   Overall Unit Performance Monitors

N/A

Category II.   Departmental Performance Monitors

Subcategory B.   Performance of Specific Departmental Functions Involving Direct Patient Care

- Capability of nursing personnel to recognize and appropriately report abnormal pulmonary function tests and abnormal blood, pH and serum electrolyte values

- Timeliness of nursing interventions to assure that patients' nutritional needs are met

- Clarity and timeliness of nurses' communication to patients regarding:

  -immediate environment
  -machinery that is or will be used
  -unit routine

- Appropriateness and timeliness of nursing interventions to reorient or maintain orientation of patients

- Completeness and accuracy of nurses' knowledge about special drugs administered in the unit

- Appropriateness of nursing judgments regarding the use of special drugs (eg, epinephrine, dopamine and nitroglycerine drips)

- Accuracy of nurses' interpretations of EKG strips

- Appropriateness and timeliness of nursing interventions to maintain patients' musculoskeletal functioning

- Accuracy and timeliness of care of invasive lines, including:

  -changing solutions at designated intervals (eg, q 24 h)
  -changing IV tubing at designated intervals (eg, q 48 h)
  -changing op-site dressings at designated intervals (eg, q 3-5 days)
  -changing Swan-Ganz/arterial line tubing at designated intervals (eg, q 48 h)

- Competence of nursing personnel in handling equipment during invasive procedures

- Accuracy of staff nurses' performance of specialized procedures, such as:

  -IABP
  -ICP
  -insertion and care of arterial lines

- Adherence to specified medical and nursing protocols for patients with neurological impairment, such as:

  -use of artificial tears
  -position change q 2 h
  -administration of antacids

- Appropriateness and timeliness of nurses' referrals to social services for family counseling during an infant's stay in the special care unit

- Adequacy of time for parent/infant interaction during an infant's stay in the special care unit

- Capability of parents upon discharge of an infant from a neonatal special care unit to use monitoring equipment and interpret monitoring data

Category II. Departmental Performance Monitors

Subcategory C. Availability, Distribution and Appropriateness of Use of Departmental Resources

- Availability of unit coverage by code-certified RNs on each shift

- Appropriateness of assignment of float personnel/registry personnel

- Assignment of nursing personnel to special care units who do not meet criteria for critical care nurses

- Appropriateness of reassignment of special care unit staff to other units based on patients' acuity levels and the number of admissions to the special care unit

- Availability of specialized equipment and supplies needed in the treatment of patients, such as:

  -oxygen
  -mechanical ventilators
  -cardiac defibrillators
  -tracheostomy, thoracostomy, thorancentesis trays
  -vascular cutdown sets
  -infusion pumps
  -laryngoscopes and endotracheal tubes
  -bed/sling weights

- Availability of respiratory therapy equipment in designated units, such as:

  -equipment to measure vital capacity and tidal and minute volumes
  -duplicate working sets of blood gas electrodes
  -oxygen analyzers
  -one functioning ventilator (vol. or pressure-set) per bed
  -humidifiers

- Availability of cannulation trays with instruments needed for inserting a prosthetic shunt in renal dialysis units

- Availability of special medications needed for patient care

- Appropriateness of physicians' requests for special equipment when more commonly used equipment is available

- Completeness and timeliness of nurses' preparation of bedside units with supplies/equipment prior to the patient's admission

Category II.   Departmental Performance Monitors

Subcategory D. Documentation

- Adequacy/accuracy of nurses' documentation of the patient's condition and progress

Category III.   User Satisfaction

- Satisfaction of patients/families (significant others) with the extent of their involvement in making informed decisions on the care that is being rendered in a special care unit

- Satisfaction of families (significant others) with the spouse support group that is sponsored by nurses in a special care unit

- Families' (significant others') satisfaction with the waiting room, including:

  -location
  -size

-physical layout
-atmosphere

- Patients' satisfaction with preparation for transfer to a general clinical unit

Category IV.   Safety Monitors

- Adherence of nursing personnel to procedures for preventing and controlling hepatitis in renal dialysis units

- Adequacy of provision for the safe disposal of infectious materials, such as:

  -contaminated dressings
  -used respiratory supplies/equipment
  -surgical instruments

- Adherence to regulations regarding the annual review and update of infection control policies and procedures

- Adherence to policies regarding the placement of infectious patients in special care units

Category V.   Quality Control Monitors

- Verification of completion of a basic critical care course by all new, permanently assigned staff in the special care unit

- Verification of CPR certification of all RNs in special care units within one month of employment

- Verification that orientees have completed a critical care skills checklist within an established time period

- Adherence to policies regarding the annual review and update of nurses' skills in performing special procedures (eg, IABP, ICP, insertion/maintenance of Swan-Ganz catheters, etc)

- Maintenance of an up-to-date professional development record which documents nurses' continuing education activities

- Verification of quarterly maintenance checks of equipment that is directly attached to patients (eg, monitors, ventilators, etc)

- Verification of semiannual maintenance checks of equipment that is not directly attached to patients

- Adequacy of daily defibrillator checks

- Maintenance of a log on the use of all battery-operated pacemakers, including:

  -date of manufacture or date of purchase
  -hours of use

- Accuracy and timeliness of checks of the water that is used for dialysis to determine its biological/chemical compatibility with acceptable renal dialysis techniques

Category VI.   Incident/Occurrence Monitors

- Rate of sepsis associated with the maintenance of arterial lines in a special care unit

Category VII.   Monitors of Patient Management and Clinical Practices of Other Departments

- Timeliness of receipt of STAT laboratory/x-ray reports

- Appropriateness and timeliness of respiratory treatments ordered for patients

- Maintenance of cleanliness/orderliness of unit by environmental services

Psychiatry-Mental Health

Category I.   Utilization Monitors

Subcategory A.   Statistical Distribution Related to Orders, Referrals and Costs

- Distribution of patients by demographics (eg, age, sex, employment status, payor status)

- Distribution of patients by acuity level and principal diagnosis

- Distribution of patients by type of concurrent medical diagnosis

- Distribution of patients by level of special observation needed (ie, continuous, q 15 min, q 30 min, q 1h, q 2h and routine)

- Readmission within a month of discharge from the unit by:

  -physician
  -primary nurse
  -type of mental illness

Category I.   Utilization Monitors

***Subcategory B.   Clinical Appropriateness and Timeliness of Admissions, Orders and
                      Referrals***

- Appropriateness of admission of patients to the acute setting when their condition does not meet admission criteria for acute intervention

- Appropriateness of outside agencies' referrals of patients to inpatient adult/pediatric psychiatric/mental health unit

- Appropriateness of referrals to the liaison nurse on psychiatric/mental health unit based on assessments made by staff in the emergency department

- Appropriateness/timeliness of referrals of mental health patients on general care units to the clinical nurse specialist in the psychiatric/mental health unit

- Appropriateness of referrals to group therapeutic activities (eg, children assigned to adult therapy groups)

- Appropriateness of the level of restrictions ordered for patients

- Appropriateness of orders for restrictions of visitors, telephone calls, mail and participation in milieu activities

- Appropriateness and timeliness of orders for seclusion of patients and for followup

- Appropriateness and timeliness of orders for restraints for patients

- Appropriateness and timeliness of orders for psychotropic medications

- Appropriateness of orders for polypharmaceutical therapy

- Appropriateness and timeliness of orders for prn medications

- Congruence of the physicians' orders with patients' multidisciplinary treatment plans

- Appropriateness and timeliness of orders for the management of patients who exhibit special problems such as:

   -suicidal ideation
   -assaultive/aggressive behavior
   -character disorders

- Appropriateness and timeliness of orders for SIP (self-injury precautions)

Category I.   Utilization Monitors

Subcategory C.   Clinicians' Use of Assessments and Recommendations Made by Staff Nurses, Clinical Nurse Specialists or Nurse Managers

- Patients' adherence to nurses' recommendations for participating in mental health/substance abuse support groups sponsored by nursing personnel

- Physicians' use of nurses' recommendations concerning patients' drug regimens

- Physicians' use of nurses' assessments to make decisions about a leave of absence/extension of hospital stay or other privileges for patients

- Physicians' use of nurses' recommendations to select group activities for patients

- Physicians' use of nurses' recommendations for managing aggressive/assaultive behavior or withdrawn patients

- Physicians' use of nurses' assessments to select the least restrictive environment for patients

Category II.   Departmental Performance Monitors

Subcategory A.   Overall Departmental Performance Monitors

- Average staff hours per patient day

- Total and average patient care hours per nurse per month for specified activities (eg, group therapy, individual consultation, etc)

- Patients' degree of attainment of treatment goals within the time specified in the treatment plan

Category II.   Departmental Performance Monitors

Subcategory B.   Performance of Specific Departmental Functions Involving Direct Patient Care

- Nurses' compliance to protocols related to the protection of patients' rights

- Adequacy of nurses' provisions for privacy of patients during the admitting process

- Completeness and timeliness of nurses' assessments of new admissions, including:

  -voluntary or committed status
  -patient's or significant other's perception of illness and the goals of therapy
  -presenting psychological signs and symptoms
  -patients's usual coping strategies
  -psychotropic drug therapy
  -patient's ability to orient him/herself to the unit
  -patient's strengths

- Completeness of nurses' biophysical assessment of patients within a specified time period after admission

- Appropriateness of nurses' determinations of the level of supervision/monitoring needed by patients

- Appropriateness of nurses' assignment of newly admitted patients to a level of restriction based on the patients' condition

- Nurses' compliance to protocols for assuring patients' right to be placed in the least restrictive environment based on their condition

- Nurses' compliance to protocols for restricting patients' privileges according to patients' assigned level of responsibility and ability

- Appropriateness and timeliness of involvement of the patient and family (significant others) in setting the goals of treatment and establishing the treatment plan

- Timeliness of nurses' updates of the plan of care for patients

- Appropriateness and timeliness of nurses' management of patients in acute crisis

- Nurses' compliance to protocols for managing patients' assaultive and aggressive behavior

- Appropriateness and timeliness of nurses' requests for placing patients in seclusion and restraints

- Appropriateness of nurses' monitoring and care of patients in seclusion and restraints

- Staff adherence to procedures for initiating and maintaining SIP for patients

- Timeliness of administration of prn medications by nursing personnel

- Timeliness and completeness of AIM (assessment of involuntary movement) by nursing personnel for patients who are receiving psychotropic drugs that may produce Parkinsonian side-effects

- Effectiveness of non-pharmacologic measures used by nurses to manage patients' behavior as an alternative to prn medication, seclusion, restraints or other restrictions

- Appropriateness of nurses' determinations of patients' need for ECT (electro-convulsive therapy)

- Appropriateness of management of therapy groups and educational sessions facilitated by nursing personnel (eg, assertiveness training, development of coping skills, stress management, etc)

- Appropriateness of recreational therapeutic activities planned by nursing personnel for patients of different age levels and/or physical limitations

- Appropriateness of the use of therapeutic role modeling by nursing personnel to instruct patients in social interaction

- Quality of nurses' therapeutic and non-therapeutic communication with patients (eg, giving advice, using judgmental statements, belittling, etc)

- Patients' knowledge of their medications following nurses' teaching

- Appropriateness and timeliness of nurses' management of elopements or "AWOL" patients

- Timeliness of nurses' authorized notification of police of patient discharge

Category II.   Departmental Performance Monitors

Subcategory C.   Availability, Distribution and Appropriateness of Use of Departmental Resources

- Appropriateness of assignment of nursing personnel based on how well patient care needs "fit" the therapeutic strengths of the staff nurse

- Adequacy of the number and mix of assigned nursing personnel so time is available for psychotherapeutic interventions by the patient's primary nurse

- Appropriateness of milieu for therapeutic management of geriatric population

- Appropriateness of milieu for therapeutic management of children

- Appropriateness of milieu for therapeutic management of manic, socially withdrawn or physically aggressive patients

- Availability of therapeutic and educational activities for patients who are restricted to the unit or denied participation in group activities

- Appropriateness and completeness of recreational equipment/facilities for substance abuse patients

- Availability of appropriate equipment for emergency care, including:

  -crash carts and defibrillators
  -suture/laceration kits
  -overdose kits

Category II.   Departmental Performance Monitors

Subcategory D.   Documentation

- Completeness and timeliness of nurses' entries on specific parts of the medical record, such as:

  -admission assessments
  -initiation of the multidisciplinary treatment plan within a specified time after
   admission
  -nursing diagnoses/patient needs' statements in progress notes

- Presence of documentation of the families' (significant others') involvement in the treatment plan

- Completeness of documentation of nurses' daily assessments of patients, including:

  -patients' ability to perform activities of daily living (ADL)
  -description of non-verbal behaviors
  -description of verbal behaviors
  -description of patients' interaction with staff and milieu

- Completeness and timeliness of the interdisciplinary team's documentation of patient's progress and status

- Completeness and timeliness of nurses' entries on the seclusion record

- Completeness and timeliness of nurses' entries on the use of restraints on patients

- Completeness and timeliness of documentation of therapies that were offered to but refused by patients

- Completeness of documentation of patients' response to specific group and educational sessions

- Completeness and timeliness of documentation of authorized searches of patients for specific objects (eg, matches, sharp objects, medications, etc) at admission and upon return from a leave of absence

- Completeness of documentation of the disposition of patient's belongings that were taken during authorized searches

- Completeness of nurses' documentation of patient knowledge of his/her medications, including:

  -name of drug(s)
  -side effects
  -risks
  -benefits

Category III.   User Satisfaction Monitors

- Families' (significant others') satisfaction with the helpfulness and effectiveness of the hospital milieu

- Patients' satisfaction with the unit's community meetings

- Families' satisfaction with family support and information meetings

Category IV.   Safety Monitors

- Adequacy of the safety of the devices in the patients' environment (eg, safety glass in windows or medicine cabinets, safety screens, etc)

- Adequacy of the system by which nurses can call for assistance in the physical management of a patient

- Adequacy of the safety of the seclusion room (eg, all areas must be visable, etc)

- Appropriateness of the disposal of used syringes/needles

Category V.   Quality Control Monitors

N/A

Category VI.   Incident/Occurrence Monitors

- Incomplete or tardy written informed consents for psychotropic drugs prescribed for patients

- Use of any psychotropic medication without documented clinical justification

- Use of the maximum dose of psychotropic drugs for more than a specified number days after admission

- Use of two or more antipsychotic medications without documented clinical justification

- Use of two or more psychotropic medications for more than a specified number of days

- Inappropriate or delayed orders for tests needed to monitor adverse/toxic effect of drugs in patients

- Inadequate checks for therapeutic blood levels of drugs administered to patients (eg, lithium)

- Maintenance of the most restrictive environment beyond a specified number of days following a patient's admission

- Use of seclusion for more than a specified number of consecutive hours

- Application of restraints more than a specified number of times in a 24-hour period

- Use of seclusion/restraints more than a specified number of times during hospitalization

- Instituting SIP or close observation of patients within a specified number of days of discharge or transfer to a less restrictive environment

- Number of patient elopements or unscheduled absences from the unit

Category VII.   Monitors of Patient Management and Clinical Practices of Other Departments

- Frequency of interdisciplinary meetings per patient or the number of times an interdisciplinary meeting was not held within 10 days of the patient's admission or once a week thereafter

- Adequacy of supervision of patients when engaged in off-unit activities

Operating Room/Recovery Room

Category I.   Utilization Monitors

Subcategory A.   Statistical Distribution Related to Orders, Referrals and Costs

- Distribution of surgical cases by:

    -type of case
    -time of day
    -day of week
    -physician
    -inpatient or outpatient status
    -type of anesthetic

- Ranking of surgeons (by service) according to their average weekly operating time

- Distribution of anesthesia time (by service) each week and month

- Total surgery hours each week and month by type of case

- Distribution of cases (by service or surgical suite) each week or month

- Operating time (by service) each week and month

- Distribution of outpatient surgery patients who are admitted by:

    -physician
    -type of case
    -type of anesthetic

- Distribution of patients admitted to the recovery room (by hour, shift, day of week) each week and month

- Average length of stay of patients in the recovery room by:

    -type of case
    -type of anesthesia
    -physician
    -inpatient/outpatient status

- Distribution of patients admitted to the recovery room (by type of anesthetic)

- Average estimated nursing costs by:

    -average patient length of stay
    -type of case
    -type of anesthetic

- Distribution of time each surgical suite is occupied by hour, day of week and week

Category I.   Utilization Monitors

Subcategory B.   Clinical Appropriateness and Timeliness of Admissions, Orders and Referrals

- Appropriateness of physicians' orders for discharge of patients from the recovery room who have not met discharge criteria

Category I.   Utilization Monitors

Subcategory C.   Clinicians' Use of Assessments and Recommendations Made by Staff Nurses, Clinical Nurse Specialists or Nurse Managers

N/A

Category II.   Departmental Performance Monitors

Subcategory A.   Overall Departmental Performance Monitors

- Ratio of daily professional and non-professional productive hours to surgery hours

- Daily non-professional hours per case

Category II.   Departmental Performance Monitors

Subcategory B.   Performance of Specific Departmental Functions Involving Direct Patient Care

- Timeliness of scheduling/adjusting cases each day by the nurse manager

- Completeness of nurses' preoperative assessment of patients, including:

  -patient's understanding of surgery
  -patient's response/experience with previous surgeries
  -patient's anxieties/concerns regarding surgery
  -allergies to medications/anesthetic agents
  -presence/absence of infection

- Adequacy of staff performance of procedures prior to surgery including:

  -surgical scrub
  -gowning
  -gloving

- Timeliness and accuracy of labeling of specimens obtained during surgery

- Adherence by nurses to procedures for procuring and administering blood

- Accuracy of staff's preparation of skin over the surgical site

- Accuracy of staff in positioning patients for surgery

- Staff competence in preparing for special operative procedures/surgical techniques, such as:

  -awareness of possible effects of special drugs used
  -awareness of possible effects of anesthetics used
  -special laboratory/x-ray procedures needed and how to respond to normal/ab-
   normal results
  -special instruments/sutures used
  -special patient positioning required
  -special safety precautions necessary

- Adherence of OR staff to procedures for the final check of the patient, including:

  -proper identification bands/tags on patient, chart and/or cart
  -written and signed consent forms
  -laboratory results

- Timeliness of nurses' notification of the family (significant others) that surgery will take longer than usual

- Adequacy of communication between the OR and recovery room concerning the patient's status

- Completeness of assessments of patients on admission to the recovery room, including:

  -vital signs
  -patency of airway
  -condition of dressings
  -condition of IVs
  -condition of drainage tubes/systems
  -pain, nausea and vomiting
  -state of consciousness
  -adequacy of peripheral circulation

- Competence of nursing personnel in the recovery room in the assessment and monitoring of patients who have received different types of anesthetics, such as:

  -spinal anesthesia
  -regional anesthesia
  -general anesthesia

- Accuracy and timeliness of performance of routine procedures in the recovery room, specifically:

  -vital signs evaluation
  -initiating coughing and deep breathing
  -airway check
  -IV check
  -"stir ups"

- Accuracy and timeliness of nurses' response to specific life-threatening conditions in the recovery room, such as:

  -hemorrhage/hypovolemia
  -aspiration
  -respiratory depression resulting from drug interaction
  -adverse reaction to/complications of anesthesia (eg, malignant hyperthermia)
  -shock

- Ability of nursing personnel in the recovery room to monitor patients with special equipment/treatment, such as:

  -compartmental pressures
  -ventilators
  -IABP
  -EKG monitors
  -subarachnoid screw for ICP monitoring

- Accuracy and timeliness of performing suctioning procedures via endotracheal/tracheostomy tubes in the recovery room

- Completeness and timeliness of instruction by nursing personnel concerning the sequence of events that will occur in the OR and the recovery room

- Accuracy and completeness of nurses' knowledge of anesthetics used in the OR, specifically:

  -classification
  -physiological action, including depth of anesthesia obtained
  -precautions
  -side-effects
  -interaction with other drugs
  -average recovery time
  -nursing implications

- Completeness/accuracy of postop nursing care and discharge instructions to same-day surgery and one-day surgery patients

Category II.   Departmental Performance Monitors

Subcategory C.   Availability, Distribution and Appropriateness of Use of Departmental Resources

- Distribution of workload among nurses and technicians

- Average RN time spent supervising other staff (ie, OR techs, aides, LPNs)

- Availability of OR staff to cover emergency cases and cases on off-shifts and weekends

- Availability of on-call coverage for the recovery room

- Utilization/nonutilization of supplies on trays (by type of operation and physician)

- Requests for special equipment by physicians when comparable equipment is available

Category II.   Departmental Performance Monitors

Subcategory D. Documentation

- Completeness of nurses' documentation of patient's peri-operative experience

- Completeness of nurses' documentation of patient's recovery room experience

Category III.   User Satisfaction Monitors

- Patients' satisfaction with their preoperative, intraoperative and postoperative stay

- Families' (significant others') satisfaction with their knowledge of the pre-operartive, intraoperative and postoperative care of the patient

- Patients' satisfaction with the knowledge of their whereabouts and condition in the OR/recovery room

- Families' (significant others') satisfaction with their knowledge of the patient's whereabouts and condition in the OR/recovery room

- Patients' satisfaction with pain control during their stay in the recovery room

- Patients'/families' (significant others') satisfaction with the outpatient surgery experience

- Physicians' satisfaction with the performance of:

  -scrub personnel
  -assistants
  -circulating nurse
  -equipment and supplies
  -cleanliness of environment

Category IV.   Safety Monitors

- Observation of routine safety measures for patients in the OR and recovery room, specifically:

  -position of siderails
  -position of patients based on the type of surgery that will be performed
  -application of restraints
  -proper identification of patients
  -locked wheels on carts

- Adherence to procedures for placing grounding plates prior to surgery

- Adherence to protocols for handling flammable gases/substances in surgical suites

- Correct identification and separation of sterile, clean and dirty areas by staff in the OR

- Adequacy and timeliness of cleaning of rooms between cases

Category V.   Quality Control Monitors

- Number of nursing personnel who are certified (CNOR-Certified Nurse of the Operating Room)

- Verification of new orientees' skills in performing specific procedures within a stated time period

- Annual verification of minimal required experience for RNs in the OR in circulating, scrub and second assistant positions

- Adherence of nursing personnel to OR/recovery room dress codes

- Accuracy of instrument and sponge counts in the OR

- Availability of sufficient scrub clothes on "off-shifts" and weekends

- Adequacy of daily checks of the effectiveness of the department's autoclave

- Verification of the integrity of the crash cart, emergency supplies and medications and functioning of the defibrillator

- Verification of weekly inventory control checks for the OR to identify and dispose of outdated items

- Verification of daily and case-by-case checks of suction equipment

- Adequacy of checks of the temperature and humidity of surgical suites

- Completeness of room setups

- Adequacy of checks of electrical equipment

- Adequacy of checks of sterilizing equipment

- Number and results of microbial checks for each surgical suite

Category VI.   Incident/Occurrence Monitors

- Lack of presurgical consultation for patients who require consultation according to institutional policy

- Inaccurate sponge, needle and instrument counts (by physician, circulating nurse and/or surgical suite)

- Omissions of needle, sponge or instrument counts as required by hospital policy

- Lapses in sterile technique (by type of procedure, physician and surgical suite)

- Infection rate of surgical wounds (by physician, surgical suite, type of surgery)

- Adverse conditions that arise during surgery or in the recovery room, such as:

  -cardiac arrest
  -respiratory arrest
  -acute myocardial infarction
  -neurological damage
  -death
  -other

- Adverse results/injury resulting from intubation

- Adverse results of anesthesia (by type of result, anesthesiologist or nurse anesthetist and type of anesthesia)

- Return to the OR for repair or removal of an organ or body part that was damaged in surgery

- Surgical procedures to repair a laceration, tear, puncture or perforation of an organ subsequent to the performance of an invasive procedure

- Errors in surgery (eg, incorrect procedure performed/procedure performed on the wrong patient/unplanned removal or repair of an organ or body part)

- Patient injury during transfer to or from the OR or recovery room

- Discovery of a foreign object or material during or after a surgical procedure

- Patient burns resulting from equipment that was used during a surgical procedure

- Patients who were released form the recovery room but did not meet discharge criteria

- Patients who were released from the recovery room but had not been evaluated by an anesthesiologist

- Outpatient surgery patients who were admitted to the hospital within 7 days after surgery (by physician, type of case, type of anesthetic)

- Complications of outpatient surgery

- Episodes of incomplete written informed consent for surgery distributed by:

  -number of incomplete consent forms
  -inconsistency between written consent and surgical procedure performed
  -number of patients who have questions about surgery after arrival in the OR
  -lack of documentation of informed consent in physicians' progress notes

Category VII.   Monitors of Patient Management and Clinical Practices of Other Departments

- Adequacy/completeness of information given to the nursing staff in the OR about emergency cases, including:

  -patient's name
  -physician's name
  -present location of patient
  -surgical procedure to be done
  -time of surgical procedure
  -disposition of family (significant others)
  -special equipment needed for surgery

- Adequacy/completeness of information given to the nursing staff in the OR about C-sections, including:

  -presence of fetal distress
  -breach presentation
  -emergent or "STAT" procedure

- Episodes of incomplete preoperative checklists by:

  -number of incomplete forms in each unit and the type of omission
  -number of surgeries delayed, postponed or canceled due to incomplete preoperative checklists
  -time lost due to delays, postponements or cancellations of surgery due to incomplete preoperative checklists

- Failure of clinical unit personnel to identify and report risk factors about patients prior to their arrival in the OR, such as:

  -obesity
  -hepatitis
  -low Hgb, Hct or abnormal blood cell levels
  -low potassium or other abnormal electrolyte levels
  -extraordinary allergies

- Time lost in the OR due to lack of appropriate information/therapy available for a patient (eg, failure of unit to send necessary medications with patient)

- Timeliness of receipt of x-ray reports

- Timeliness of room setup for each case

- Timeliness of start of cases or the number of late cases (by physician and/or surgical suite)

- Timeliness of administration of anesthesia (by anesthesiologist and surgical suite)

Emergency Department

Category I.   Utilization Monitors

Subcategory A.   Statistical Distribution Related to Orders, Referrals and costs

- Distribution of patients who use the emergency room by:

  -time of day/day of week
  -age
  -sex
  -payor status
  -diagnosis/DRG
  -address/zip code
  -level of acuity

- Utilization of emergency nurse practitioner (by number of patients served, acuity level and admitting/discharge diagnosis)

- Utilization of special treatment rooms (by time of day, day of week, patient acuity level, average length of stay in the room and discharge diagnosis)

- Number of patients/families who need grief/bereavement counseling, crisis counseling or social service referral

Category I.   Utilization Monitors

Subcategory B.   Clinical Appropriateness and Timeliness of Admissions, Orders and Referrals

- Appropriateness/timeliness of transfers to the emergency department from other institutions, including:

  -total number of transfers per month
  -transferring physician
  -transferring institution
  -discharge diagnosis of physician in referring institution
  -physician responsible for receiving the patient
  -condition of the patient on arrival from the transferring agency
  -type of case (eg, critical care, medical-surgical, etc)
  -availability of orders at the time of patient's arrival

- Timeliness of physician's response to notification of patient's arrival in the emergency department

- Timeliness of discharge of patients from the emergency department

- Appropriateness and timeliness of patient transfer to another institution from the emergency room, including:

  -total number of monthly transfers

-condition of the patient at the time of the transfer
-discharge diagnosis
-transferring physician
-receiving agency
-receiving physician (if known)
-method of transfer

Category I.   Utilization Monitors

Subcategory C.   Clinicians' Use of Nursing Assessments and Recommendations Made by Staff Nurses, Clinical Nurse Specialists or Nurse Managers

N/A

Category II.   Departmental Performance Monitors

Subcategory A.   Overall Departmental Performance Monitors

- Time spent by "Express Care" patients waiting for treatment

- Through-put time of patients entering the emergency department by status of patients, eg:

    -urgent
    -emergent
    -non-emergent

Category II.   Departmental Performance Monitors

Subcategory B.   Performance of Specific Departmental Functions Involving Direct Patient Care

- Adequacy of communication between nurses in the emergency department and ambulance EMTs and nurses outside the institution, including:

    -the exchange of essential information related to the patient's complaints
    -the pertinence and clarity of communication
    -the quality of communication regarding telemetry

- Appropriateness of radio directions given by nursing personnel in the emergency department

- Timeliness of nursing assessment of patients entering the emergency department by status of patient, eg:

    -urgent
    -emergent
    -non-emergent

- Appropriateness of nurses' case management of patients who have been transported by air to the emergency department

- Appropriateness and accuracy of nurse(s)' triage judgments regarding:

  -assignment of patients to a priority rating
  -assignment of patients to a nurse based on the patient's needs, the nurse's expertise and current workload
  -accuracy of requests for initial diagnostic studies

- Competence of nursing personnel in the initial management of specific types of emergencies, such as:

  -head injuries
  -poisonings
  -gunshot/stab wounds
  -animal bites
  -major trauma
  -impending MI (myocardial infarction)

- Competence of nursing personnel in the management of pediatric emergencies

- Appropriateness of treatment of pregnant women by:

  -trimester of pregnancy
  -type of medication prescribed in the emergency department
  -discharge diagnosis
  -timing of emergency therapy
  -type of surgery performed in the emergency department

- Appropriateness and timeliness of nurses' management of suspected victims of rape, sexual molestation and/or child/spouse abuse

- Appropriateness and timeliness of nurses' management of patients who have known or suspected contagion (eg, AIDS, radioactive contamination, etc)

- Appropriateness of nurses' management of patients who are mentally ill or under the influence of drugs or alcohol

- Appropriateness of physical management of psychiatric-mental health patients by nursing personnel in the emergency department

- Appropriateness of care rendered to an unemancipated minor who is not accompanied by a parent or guardian or to any unaccompanied unconscious patient

- Competence of nursing personnel in performing critical procedures mandated by JCAH, such as:

  -ACLS
  -parenteral administration of fluids, electrolytes and blood
  -wound care
  -management of sepsis

-initial burn care

-initial management of injuries to the extremities

-initial management of injuries to the CNS

-recognition of and attention to the social and psycholological needs of patients and families

- Competence of nursing staff in the performance of the following specialized skills:

-auto-transfusion technique

-setup of "thumper"

-setup for a thoracotomy

-setup for IABP

-setup for pacemaker insertion

-setup for insertion of Swan-Ganz line

-setup for burr hole insertion

-setup for insertion of tongs

- Adherence of nursing personnel to written protocols for the following:

-starting two IV solutions

-applying mast trousers

-administering oxygen

-stabilizing a fracture

-controlling bleeding

- Timeliness of nurses' administration of tetanus immunization to patients for whom it is indicated

- Appropriateness and timeliness of notification of next of kin, pastoral care and/or medical examiner when a patient dies in the emergency department

- Accuracy of completion of body release form by nurses when a death occurs in the emergency department

- Appropriateness and timeliness of the release of information and materials to police or health authorities

- Completeness and timeliness of patient information reported from the emergency department by nursing personnel to another department (eg, admitting, operating room, radiology, etc) concerning the status of a patient

- Compliance of emergency department personnel with written transfer protocols

- Degree of patients' adherence to followup instructions given by nursing personnel in the emergency department

Category II.   Departmental Performance Monitors

Subcategory C.   Availability, Distribution and Appropriateness of Use of Departmental Resources

- Availability and effectiveness of flexible schedules of nursing personnel (ie, 10-hr and 12-hr shifts) to cover peak utilization times

- Availability of needed equipment and supplies, such as:

    -cardiac monitors

    -thoracotomy trays

    -tracheostomy trays

    -pleural and pericardial drainage sets

    -emergency obstetrical packs

    -laryngoscopes and endotracheal tubes

    -vascular cutdown sets

    -infusion pumps

- Degree of loss of equipment to inpatient care areas

Category II.   Departmental Performance Monitors

Subcategory D.   Documentation

- Completeness and timeliness of nurses' documentation of radio orders during patient's transport to the department

- Adequacy of the control register maintained in the emergency department

- Completeness and timeliness of nurses' documentation of patient visits to the emergency room, including:

    -patient identification

    -method of arrival

    -pertinent history of illness or injury

    -vital signs

    -emergency care rendered prior to arrival in the department

    -clinical observations, especially the response to treatment

    -discharge instructions given to the patient or family (significant others)

- Appropriateness of nurses' documentation of the site of medication administration and the patient's response to the medication

Category III.   User Satisfaction Monitors

- Patients' satisfaction with the nursing services given in the emergency department

- Patients'/families' satisfaction with timeliness of nursing care

- Patients'/families' satisfaction with the timeliness and completeness of information given about the patient throughout treatment, including

  -patient informed of the cause of delay
  -family informed of patient's status when not with the patient

- Patients' satisfaction with the clarity and timeliness of the information given him/her about diagnostic findings and treatment regimin

Category IV.   Safety Monitors

- Adherence of nursing staff to procedures for identifying patients for tests and treatments

- Adequacy of identification and isolation of patients who enter the emergency department with an infectious disease

- Correct use of siderails for minors, patients with decreased alertness or possibility of seizures

- Adequacy of equipment checks for proper grounding

Category V.   Quality Control Monitors

- Verification of ACLS completion by all RNs within six months of assignment to the emergency department

- Verification of completion of critical care classes by nursing personnel within six months of assignment to the emergency department

- Verification of ATLS (advanced trauma life support) completion within nine months of assignment to the emergency department

- Verification of recertification for ACLS of each nurse in the emergency department every two years

- Verification annually of nurses' maintenance of acceptable skill levels for common procedures performed in the department

- Verification of routine maintenance checks of equipment needed in the emergency department, such as:

  -oxygen equipment
  -ventilators
  -defibrillators

-monitoring equipment (eg, cardiac, respiratory, neurological, etc)
-suction equipment

- Adequacy of inventory of required supplies including:

  -turnover rate of items
  -disposal of outdated materials

- Thoroughness of crash cart checks during each shift

Category VI.   Incident/Occurrence Monitors

- Patients who were erroneously dismissed because their symptoms did not appear to constitute a real emergency

- Patients who received treatment before consent for treatment had been obtained (by age and acuity level)

- Transfers of unstabilized patients to or from the department

- Patients who returned to the emergency department within 48 hours of discharge

- Deaths during patients' stay in emergency department

- Deaths of patients within 7 days of discharge from the emergency department

- Misdiagnosis of patients by physicians in the emergency department

- Discrepancies between the discharge diagnosis and laboratory/radiology reports

- Patients who were not seen by a physician during a visit to the emergency department

- Treatment of patients in the emergency department by physicians via telephone

- Complications from a specified procedure/therapy (eg, tracheostomy, endotracheal intubation, cardiac massage, etc)

- Inappropriate chemotherapeutic management of psychiatric-mental health patients in the emergency department

Category VII.   Monitors of Patient Management and Clinical Practices of Other Departments

- Adequacy of the followup care mechanism (ie, the mechanism whereby emergency department records are made available to followup agencies

- Turnaround time for x-rays, laboratory studies

- Timeliness of notification of sexual assault counselor after report of incident

- Appropriateness, accuracy and timeliness of notification of patient of X-ray/laboratory results after discharge from the emergency department

Bibliography

Artinian B, O'Connor F and Brock R: Comparing past and present nursing productivity. *Nursing Management* 15(10):50-53, October 1984.

Barness S and Long C: Perioperative Nursing. *AORN Journal* 39(4):609-615, March 1984.

Baum J: Emergency hospital care: Issues of treatment and liability. *Medical Malpractice Cost Containment Journal* 1(1):27-31, Spring (April) 1979.

Bennett G: Communicating with the hospital infection control practitioner: Can it benefit me? *Occupational Health Nursing*, 20-22, January 1983.

Braulick R, Coronado J, Heil E, Burt M and Lutonsky R: On the scene: Audie L. Murphy Memorial Veterans Hospital. *Nursing Administration Quarterly*, 15-33, Spring 1983.

Brenner L and Jessee W: Delays in diagnosis: A problem for quality assurance. *Quality Review Bulletin* 9(11):337-344, November 1983.

Buechler D: Code blue evaluation. *Nursing Management* 13(5):25-28, May 1982.

Clausen C: Staff RN: A discharge planner for every patient. *Nursing Management* 15(11):58-61, November 1984.

Coleman J and Smith D: DRGs: Opportunity or crisis? *Pediatric Nursing*, 321-323, September/October 1984.

Conway C and Johnston P: Integrating clinical and management systems in nursing. *Hospital Topics*, 14-17, May/June 1984.

Dale R and Mable R: Nursing Classification System: Foundation for personnel planning and control. *The J of Nursing Adm*, 10-14, February 1983.

del Bueno D: Doing the right thing· Nurses' ability to make clinical decisions. 7-11, Autumn 1983.

DeMilliano M: 8 common charting mistakes to avoid. *Nursing Life*, 30-32, May/June 1984.

Distel L: A nursing quality assurance investigation of orthopedic patient care. *Quality Review Bulletin*, 20-22, October 1982.

Fife D, Soloman P and Stanton M: A risk/falls program: Code orange for success. *Nursing Management* 15(11):50-53, November 1984.

Forehand J: Nursing quality assurance study of code blue drills. *Quality Review Bulletin*, 117-119, April 1984.

Franz J: Challenge for nursing: Hiking productivity without lowering quality of care. *Modern Healthcare*, 60-68, September 1984.

Fray C: An accountability - classification instrument for orthopaedic patients. *The J of Nursing Adm,* 32-28, July-August 1984.

Friss L and White M: Productivity in nursing. *Topics in Health Care Financing,* 83-104.

Gay P: Get it in writing. *Nursing Management* 14(3):32-35.

Goplerud E and Finger J: Quality assurance in a CMHC: A program to use underutilized resources. *Quality Review Bulletin* 10(5):150-152, May 1984.

Hagey R and McDonough P: The problem of professional labeling. *Nursing Outlook,* 151-157, May/June 1984.

Halloran E: Staffing assignment: By task or by patient. *Nursing Management* 14(8):16-18.

Hancock W, Flynn P, DeRosa S, Walter P and Conway C: A cost and staffing comparison of an all-RN staff and team nursing. *Nursing Administration Quarterly,* 45-55, Winter 1984.

Hanson R: Managing human resources. *The J of Nursing Adm,* 17-23, December 1982.

Heister, Johnson B and Trimberger L: ED standards and audit criteria. *Journal of Emergency Nursing,* 83-38, April, 1982.

Herzog T: Productivity: Fighting the battle of the budget. *Nursing Management* 16(1):30-34, January 1985.

How much does nursing care really cost? *Am J of Nursing,* 942-943, July 1984.

Innes E and Turman W: Evaluation of patient falls. *Quality Review Bulletin,* 30-35, February 1983.

Joint Commission of Accreditation of Hospitals: *Accreditation Manual for Hospitals* (Chicago, Joint Commission on Accreditation of Hospitals) 1985.

Joseph E: *Risk Management in Mental Health.* (Chicago: Care Communications, Inc.) 1981.

Joseph E and Beck E: *Quality Assurance/Risk Management: The Nurse's Perspective.* (Chicago: Care Communications, Inc.) 1981.

Joseph E, DeVet C and Dehn T: *The Monitoring Sourcebook, Vol. 1: Radiology, Pharmacy, Clinical Laboratory.* (Chicago: Care Communications, Inc.) 1985.

Joseph E, Shannon K and Svendson, G: *A DRG and Prospective Pricing Action Plan for Nursing.* (Chicago: Care Communications, Inc.) 1983.

Joseph V and Jones S: Managerial briefs. *Nursing Management* 15(12):20-23, December 1984.

Lang D: Prospective quality assurance. *Quality Review Bulletin,* 143-145, May 1984.

Lee A: How DRGs will affect your hospital—and you. *RN,* 71-81, May 1984.

Lillesand K and Korff S: Nursing process evaluation: A quality assurance tool. *Nursing Administration Quarterly,* 9-14, Spring 1983.

Meier P and Todd C: Four-day, forty-hour workweek for neonatal intensive care nurses. *JOGN Nursing* (Supplement), 89s-95s, May/June 1983.

Meisenheimer C: Incorporating JCAH standards into a quality assurance program. *Nursing Administration Quarterly,* 1-8, Spring 1983.

Mohr B and Joseph E: *The Role of Nurses in Risk Management.* (Chicago: Care Communications, Inc.) 1981.

Morrison S: Monitoring decubitus ulcers: A monthly survey method. *Quality Review Bulletin* 10(4):112-117, April 1984.

On the scene: Quality control circles at Barnes Hospital. *Nursing Administration Quarterly,* 23-46, Spring 1982.

Perry S: Evaluating nursing care through medical record review. *Journal of AMRA,* 28-31, December 1984.

Rasmusen L: A screening tool promotes early discharge planning. *Nursing Management,* 39-43, May 1984.

Robbins D: Dealing with grief and bereavement in the emergency department. *Journal of Emergency Nursing* 9(4):228-233, July/August 1983.

Rogers J, Haring O and Goetz J: Changes in patient attitudes following the implementation of a medical information system. *Quality Review Bulletin,* March 1984.

Schulmerich C: Implementing staggered twelve-hour shifts for ED nurses. *Journal of Emergency Nursing,* 127-131.

Shukla R: Nursing care structures and productivity. *Hospital & Health Services Administration,* 45-58, Nov/Dec 1982.

Smith C: DRGs - Making them work for you. *Nursing 85,* 35-41, January.

Smith H and Reid R: Short and long run management strategies for DRGs. *Hospital Topics,* 4-7, 39-40, 48, May/June 1984.

Stearns G, Fox L, Imbiorski W and Joseph E: *Solutions: Integrate, simplify, monitor quality assurance/risk management activities.* (Chicago: Care Communications, Inc.) 1981.

Swartzbeck E: The problems of falls in the elderly. *Nursing Management* 14(12):35-38, December, 1983.

Thee K and Obrecht W: Using a patient routing list to document preoperative instruction. *Quality Review Bulletin,* 149-152, May 1984.

The Nurses Association of the American College of Obstetricians and Gynecologists: *Standards for Obstetric, Gynecologic, and Neonatal Nursing.* (2nd ed.) Washington, D.C., The Nurses Association of the American College of Obstetricians and Gynecologists, 1981.

The Nursing Management Report. *Nursing & Health Care,* 199-203, April.

Thornton L: Nursing Algorithms. *The J of Nursing Adm,* 11-15, January 1985.

Torrez Sister M: Systems approach to staffing. *Nursing Management* 14(5):54-58.

Villeneuve M: The patient compliance puzzle. *Nursing Management* 13(5):54-56, May 1982.

Vogel L, Wicker M, Harlan J and Thorup, Jr. O: Use of nursing hours in measuring hospital productivity. *Nursing Administration Quarterly,* 90-97, Winter 1984.

Walts L and Blair F: Making quality assurance work in the emergency department. *Journal of Emergency Nursing* 9(1):59-64, February 1983.

Watson P: The effects of short-term postoperative counseling on cancer/ostomy patients. *Cancer Nursing,* 21-28, February 1983.

Whybrow A: Management Survival Kit - Monitoring the services. *Nursing Mirror,* 45-46, December 15, 1982.

Widhalm A and Anderson L: Emergency nurse practitioners: Motivators, barriers and autonomy in role performance. *Journal of Emergency Nursing,* Pg. 67-74.

Zoebelein E, Levy M and Greenwald R: The effect of quality assurance review on implementation of an automatic stop-order policy. *Quality Review Bulletin,* 12-17, August 1982.

Zwicke D, Bobzien W and Wagner E: Triage nurse decisions: A prospective study. *Journal of Emergency Nursing,* 132-137.

Worksheets

Unit/Department Monitoring Profile

CATEGORY: UTILIZATION MONITORS

Subcategory: Statistical Distribution of·Orders, Referrals and Costs

CURRENT TOPICS BEING MONITORED	CONTINUE?		ALTERNATIVE/ ADDITIONAL TOPICS	PRIORITY?	
	Yes	No		Yes	No

Unit/Department Monitoring Profile

CATEGORY: UTILIZATION MONITORS

Subcategory: Clinical Appropriateness and Timeliness of Admissions, Orders and Referrals

CURRENT TOPICS BEING MONITORED	CONTINUE?		ALTERNATIVE/ ADDITIONAL TOPICS	PRIORITY?	
	Yes	No		Yes	No

Unit/Department Monitoring Profile

CATEGORY: UTILIZATION MONITORS

Subcategory: Clinicians' Use of Assessments and Recommendations Made by Staff Nurses, Clinical Nurse Specialists or Nurse Managers

CURRENT TOPICS BEING MONITORED	CONTINUE?		ALTERNATIVE/ ADDITIONAL TOPICS	PRIORITY?	
	Yes	No		Yes	No

Unit/Department Monitoring Profile

CATEGORY: DEPARTMENTAL PERFORMANCE MONITORS

Subcategory: Overall Departmental Performance Monitors

CURRENT TOPICS BEING MONITORED	CONTINUE?		ALTERNATIVE/ ADDITIONAL TOPICS	PRIORITY?	
	Yes	No		Yes	No

Unit/Department Monitoring Profile

CATEGORY: DEPARTMENTAL PERFORMANCE MONITORS

Subcategory: Performance of Specific Departmental Functions Involving Direct Patient Care

CURRENT TOPICS BEING MONITORED	CONTINUE?		ALTERNATIVE/ ADDITIONAL TOPICS	PRIORITY?	
	Yes	No		Yes	No

Unit/Department Monitoring Profile

CATEGORY: DEPARTMENTAL PERFORMANCE MONITORS

Subcategory: Availability, Distribution and Appropriateness of Use of Departmental Resources

CURRENT TOPICS BEING MONITORED	CONTINUE?		ALTERNATIVE/ ADDITIONAL TOPICS	PRIORITY?	
	Yes	No		Yes	No

Unit/Department Monitoring Profile

CATEGORY: DEPARTMENTAL PERFORMANCE MONITORS

Subcategory: Documentation

CURRENT TOPICS BEING MONITORED	CONTINUE?		ALTERNATIVE/ ADDITIONAL TOPICS	PRIORITY?	
	Yes	No		Yes	No

Copyright © Care Communications, Inc.

Unit/Department Monitoring Profile

CATEGORY: SAFETY MONITORS

Subcategory:

CURRENT TOPICS BEING MONITORED	CONTINUE?		ALTERNATIVE/ ADDITIONAL TOPICS	PRIORITY?	
	Yes	No		Yes	No

Copyright © Care Communications, Inc.

Unit/Department Monitoring Profile

CATEGORY: QUALITY CONTROL MONITORS

Subcategory:

CURRENT TOPICS BEING MONITORED	CONTINUE?		ALTERNATIVE/ ADDITIONAL TOPICS	PRIORITY?	
	Yes	No		Yes	No

Unit/Department Monitoring Profile

CATEGORY: INCIDENT/OCCURRENCE MONITORS

Subcategory:

CURRENT TOPICS BEING MONITORED	CONTINUE?		ALTERNATIVE/ ADDITIONAL TOPICS	PRIORITY?	
	Yes	No		Yes	No

Unit/Department Monitoring Profile

CATEGORY: MONITORS OF PATIENT MANAGEMENT AND CLINICAL PRACTICES OF OTHER DEPARTMENTS

Subcategory:

CURRENT TOPICS BEING MONITORED	CONTINUE?		ALTERNATIVE/ ADDITIONAL TOPICS	PRIORITY?	
	Yes	No		Yes	No